Neal —
To my
Sports + Lunch
"Buddy"
Happy Reading!!
Maddy

Johnny Run Lately

The Life and Adventures of a Latter Day Sprint Champion

John Hurd

ISBN 978-1-63490-513-8

Published by BookLocker.com, Inc., Bradenton, Florida, U.S.A.

Printed on acid-free paper.

BookLocker.com, Inc.
2015

First Edition

Dedication

To my sisters, Bobbie Hurd Davis 1925-1998,
and Billie Hurd Newman 1929-2013.

Acknowledgements

To my loving wife, Sandy – my Best Friend, my supporter, my cheerleader, my PR person, and my motivator, who has been with me 100% every step of the way, especially when I was ready to give up. Sandy helped me get started with the book, did most of the creative work, designed the cover, wrote part of the book, and helped with the editing. Thank you, Sandy.

To my sister Jo Hurd Lowery and brother Walker Hurd, who, along with Bobbie and Billie, have contributed so much to who and what I am.

To my son, Kevin, who wrote in this book about his experience being with me at the National Games in 2013.

To our friend, Iris Lawrence, whose suggestions for the text on the back cover reduced it from three rambling paragraphs to one that that made sense to me.

There are a lot of people mentioned or pictured within these pages, who appear to have no connection to my story about my running hobby, but all of them do. In one way or another, these are some of the family members and friends and competitors who have given their love and support and encouragement to me. This book, then, is a tribute to them, and my way of broadcasting a heart-felt "thank you all" for all that you have done for, and meant to, me.

Thank you all, and please know that I appreciate and love all of you.

PROLOGUE

As a boy growing up, I missed out on a lot of fun – and I should add, probably some degree of trouble. I attribute this to three things: I was very, very small, I was painfully shy, and I came from a home that had very little means. I was the first boy, the fourth of five kids, aged nine, seven, five, three, and two months when my mother was widowed.

So, what *did* I have? I had good health, a good mind, and I lived in a house full of love, with a mother that would have given her very life for any of her kids. And she eventually did. We had relatives, from Mother's side and Daddy's side, who were always there for us, especially during those growing up years.

Did I eventually overcome these three "handicaps?" Yes, at least to the extent and beyond that which I would have believed at the time.

In the early grades in school, I had two attributes that kept me from being a complete dud. I could read aloud well in class, and I was good at arithmetic at the chalk board. I would sit and wait impatiently while each child took their turn to read, and by the time it was my turn to read my mouth would be so dry you could have struck a match on it. In arithmetic class the teacher would have several of us at the chalk board at one time, so when she gave us an arithmetic problem to do, it was a race. I absolutely had to win, and I usually did. My real thrill would come when one of the parents was visiting. That was how I got my strokes.

My high school of about 1,100 kids began in the tenth grade. In my first year I was 5 feet 0 inches tall, and weighed 92 pounds. The team sports coaches didn't seem to be begging me to come and try out for their teams. There was not much I could do about that, but by graduation time I had made it all the way to 5 feet 6 ½ inches, and weighed 124 pounds. By the end of college, at age 24, I was 5 feet 8 (if I held the tape) and 136 pounds. By then I had worked full time for a year or so, and served a two year active duty hitch in Uncle Sugar's Navy, during the Korean War. There still didn't seem to be much point in trying to be a jock at that time.

It may not have been entirely true when I said there was not much I could do about my size. Mother taught me very early in life that smoking would stunt my growth, and drinking would be bad for my mind and for my overall health. So, except for my one and only package of cigarettes at age five (more about that in Chapter One), and a small glass of what I call sissy wine that I enjoy before dinner at home now, I never took up either habit. I still don't know what hard liquor or even beer tastes like.

During those early school years, including high school, the shyness, my diminutive size, and the lack of funds for dressing and going places somewhat hampered my social life. I did get by and still maintained an optimistic spirit throughout. But by the time I got out of school, I decided that enough was enough. I had to do something.

I started reading self-help books long before it was popular to admit that you read such things. I read *How to Win Friends and Influence People*, *Psycho Cybernetics*, *The Magic of*

Thinking Big, The Magic of Believing, Think and Grow Rich and on and on. There was no real "aha" that "changed my life," but little by little the layers began to have an effect on my beginning to believe in myself.

Why am I telling you all this stuff about my life? To give you hope. If you've had anything in your life that you wish you had done, or hope you can do "some day," I want you to understand that there is still time for you.

So please turn to the next page, and come with me while I share things about me and my experiences, some of which will be revealed for the first time. I hope you enjoy it.

John Hurd
Age 83

Contents

1
Let's Start at the Beginning...

The leaves were turning red and gold and a chill wind was blowing like a gale. My family lived in a tiny town on the Tennessee bank of the Mississippi River, 10 miles from the nearest light bulb and right on the state line between Tennessee and Missouri, thus the name "Tennemo," where I was born. The maps show a population under 250, the smallest dot they use. It is so tiny that my birth certificate shows Miston, the other tiny town where Cuddin Oscar and his wife Zettie lived. (When a cousin was from an older generation, we addressed them by that title, which rhymes with sudden.) The house we lived in was a small frame house up on stilts, as sometimes the river would flood. The tar paper on the walls did its best to keep the wind from coming through the cracks. Living up that high made it seem even colder on this particular night.

Most of my family were farmers by trade, and they had been working all day in the fields. Cousin Zettie remarked "I sure hope Bill don't send for me tonight, I'm so tired." You see, Mother was pregnant with me and about to deliver. She was just called "Bill" by the family, but her real name was Mary Willie Reeks before she married my father, Elbert Eugene "Jack" Hurd.

It was the night of October 20, 1931, when Mother went into labor and Daddy couldn't get the car started, so he left to go over to Cousin Oscar's house to get help in getting a doctor. I arrived on October 21st, about 10 minutes after midnight, about thirty minutes before the doctor and Daddy came.

There were just me and Mother and three sisters, ages five, three and one, there at home together. Mother said I was the coldest and hungriest of all of her children. I still do much better in warm weather.

There were eventually five of us: my oldest sister Bobbie, then Jo and then Billie (born on Halloween, three days after Black Monday, which kicked off the Great Depression), and then me. Each of us came about two years apart, but my little brother, Walker, came along three years after I did. Mother said Daddy named all of us, and since we were a farming family, he probably wanted boys, so he named all three of the girls with boys' names. However, he had a nickname for each of us. I don't remember Bobbie's, but Jo was called Dago because she loved spaghetti. Billie was Runt, and I was Jabbo. Maybe I actually jabbered a lot in my "Daddy" years, but later I became the shyest person in the history of mankind. Or maybe it was because of my lightning fast left jab. Or maybe not. Walker was Pedro. I don't understand that one either, because he was too young to eat tacos. As for parents' names, in the South we didn't have moms and dads; we had mothers and daddies, or mommas and poppas. And they, like all other grown-ups and people of authority, were addressed as ma'am or sir. No exceptions.

I refer to that time as my "Daddy" years, because barely two months after Walker was born, Daddy, along with another man, was struck and killed by a car while helping someone get his wagon out of a ditch on a rainy night. That left Mother with five kids, ages nine years to two months, and a $54 monthly government check from an injury Daddy sustained in World War I. The closest I came to having a grandparent was

Mother's mother, who died in the 1918 flu epidemic, 13 years to the day before I was born. Mother gave up a scholarship to college to look after her three younger siblings: Louise, Muriel and John.

My memories of Daddy were few but vivid and all good. From the floor up, he looked like a giant. His World War I Army discharge papers listed him as 5 ft. 5½ inches. On my third birthday he tried to tell me "Jabbo's three years old." But I had learned that Jabbo was two years old, so we argued over that with "Jabbo two years old." He would let me drive the horses and wagon in the field and even on the roads. He taught me to say "gee" to turn right and "haw" to turn left, and "whoa" to stop, hence the expression "They don't gee and haw so well together," meaning they think in different directions.

The relatives wanted Mother to split us up into different families, but she would have none of that. We did, however, receive a lot of help from all the relatives over the next few years. We spent time scattered among Mother's siblings and Daddy's aunts. At age four we moved to the town of Dyersburg, Tennessee and lived for a short while with Mother's sister, Aunt Louise Condrey, Uncle Ervin and their daughter Glenda, our only first cousin. Here we finally got electricity and running water and an indoor bathroom.

I never knew where it originated, but I was extremely bashful, and would go to any length to avoid calling attention to myself. I can remember sitting at the dinner table with the family, just waiting and hoping that someone would offer me another biscuit, or another serving of beans. If the offer didn't come, I didn't get it. Even earlier than that, I remember being at Uncle John Reeks's house (Mother's only brother). They were crowded around me trying to give me a penny if I would just say "please." But the word would not come and I never did get the penny. It was like that all my growing-up years. I just wouldn't ask anybody for anything.

By 1936 all six of us had moved into a two family house in Dyersburg, where each family had three rooms and we shared a common bathroom off the back porch. It had an overhead light bulb with a pull down string, and a commode. The only other source of water was a faucet in the kitchen sink, and it was cold. To bathe we heated water in pans on the wood-burning cook stove and brought a wash tub into the kitchen. The rent was initially $9.00 per month. That's not a typo; it was nine dollars a month.

Next door were Mr. and Mrs. Jernigan, Doris, Polly, and Gene. Gene and I were instantly the best of friends, and remained so until he passed away in 2012. We played football, cowboys, and croquet and made up games all in the lot between our houses. In the summer we would have foot races barefoot on the sidewalk. Gene usually won, because my entire body was barely taller than his legs. When his brother would visit from Memphis (he was 19 or so, and I thought he was so mature), he'd get the boxing gloves out, and work my corner. Gene usually won those too, because besides being so much taller than I was, he was also a southpaw.

We were never poor, we just didn't have any money. The Jernigans had an electric refrigerator, a car, a telephone, a radio, a bathtub with hot water, and most important, they had a daddy. During the nine years we were in that house, we finally did get a plug-in icebox (refrigerator), a telephone and a radio. Televisions were not around till much, much later. I first heard of them in a newsreel at the picture show when I was about twelve. They said this would be real in our homes in about ten years.

Part of the summer of 1937 we spent in Lucy, Tennessee with mother's other sister, Aunt Muriel (rhymes with curl) and Uncle Henry Walker on their farm. It was there that Uncle Henry taught me how to hold a fork, and he taught me how to smoke – or rather, how not to smoke. He was a smoker, and often he would finish a cigarette and give it to me to throw away in the front yard. I would do that, but not until I had a few puffs off of it myself. I didn't think he caught on to that.

There was another boy that I played with, and he and I got the grandiose idea of collecting cigarettes and taking the tobacco and saving it for a real smoke session the following Saturday. Well, by the time Saturday came we had the tobacco and paper, but nothing to light them with. So I got the brilliant idea of walking down to the store and charging a penny box of matches to Uncle Henry's account. Where that courage came from I'll never know. The man at the store must have ratted on me, because later that day I faced an inquisition. They had me cold. The verdict was that Uncle Henry would bring me my own package of cigarettes the next day, and we would smoke properly. I learned later that he had cleared this risky idea with Mother.

The next day I watched for him all day. Finally, he arrived and I had my own package of Old Gold cigarettes. Of course I couldn't read the label, but I did know the difference between a camel and a stack of gold coins on the packages. I thought it was a little strange, giving me a different brand that was not the same one he smoked. Anyway, we went to the next room together, where he lit my cigarette, and had one for himself. When we finished them, he stuck another one in my hand, and said "Have another." Again, I thought that was a little strange, but I was only five years old, so what the heck. About half way through that second one, Aunt Muriel came into the room to call us to supper, (we had dinner at noon and supper at dark) and screamed "Henry, what are you doing?" Actually, I wasn't very hungry by that time, and that was the last package of cigarettes I ever owned.

Mother used that strategy on me a few years later when I thought I wanted a cup of coffee. None of us in the family drank coffee, but when Cousin Oscar (Zettie's husband) came to visit, she would make coffee for him. A cup and a half of that stuff, strong and black, was all I needed. It was 25 years later before I had my next cup of coffee.

2
The Early Years

By the fall of 1937 we were all back together as a family in Dyersburg. Although we had little, we were a happy family. At supper time, after we finished, one of the girls would jump up from the table and exclaim "I'm gonna dry." I never figured out why being the one to dry the dishes was so important. They sang songs while they washed and dried the dishes and everything was happy and fun. They sang the popular songs of the time, such as *In the Mood*, *Elmer's Tune*, *Frenesi*, *Amapola*, and *After the Ball Was Over*. My sisters helped take care of me and cooked and cleaned and helped Mother. I still don't cook to this day, because they spoiled me so much.

Mother was always teaching us. The two main lessons were:

(1) If we knew something we were thinking about doing was wrong, then we were not to do it. I can still remember her saying, "I don't care if it's a bent rusty nail. If it is in someone else's yard, it is not yours, and you don't take it." I remember one day when Walker was just barely old enough to walk, Mother sent us to the grocery store for some small item. While there, Walker picked up a piece of penny candy and took it home. Mother sent both of us back to the store to pay for the candy. Between my shyness and the unusual nature of the event, it took the store manager quite a while to understand what I was trying to tell him. When I was a little older I found two $5 bills on the sidewalk. When I took the ten dollars into the house, Mother wanted to buy an ad in the newspaper to locate the person who lost it. Mr. Jernigan, next door, finally convinced her that doing that would be fruitless.

(2) We were meant to be healthy. If one of us came to Mother feeling bad, or something hurt, she might ask us "Well, where did that come from?" and we would say we didn't know. She would usually reply with, "It'll go right back there, then." She wasn't dismissing a real Illness; she just knew more about what ailed us than we did. She believed that you could think yourself into an ailment just because someone you knew had it. I believe I can honestly say that to this day I have never believed that I caught something bad from someone else. I don't remember her preaching that certain foods were bad for you, and some were good. For many years we were very fortunate to be eating at all. She believed that if God put it here for you to eat, it was good. I learned at a very early age to stay well and that good health or sickness usually originated with my thinking. Thanks to Mother, I have managed to stay healthy most of my life and my weight has not fluctuated more than five or ten pounds since I graduated from college in 1956.

Once I started to school I would occasionally do odd jobs to earn money for the Saturday picture show and a bag of popcorn. That came to a total of 15 cents. I would clean Miss Ella's chicken coop or run errands for her. I clipped a coupon from a comic book and sold $4.00 worth of garden and flower seeds to get a Red Ryder BB gun. The price in the stores was $2.95. I grew corn in my back yard and peddled it in the neighborhood from my red wagon. It sold at ten cents for three ears. I earned my first full dollar (and two cents) by picking 51 pounds of cotton, which was much more than I weighed. I even sold doughnuts door to door for a local bakery. That ended in disaster. I knocked on this one door, and two young girls told me to go upstairs and ask their mother. I neared the top of the stairs and their half-dressed mother started screaming like a banshee. I retired from my bakery sales career at a very early age.

In the summer of 1943, at age eleven, I had my first full time job. Gene's daddy arranged for Gene and me to have a job setting pins in a bowling alley. They had quit making new cars when the war started (WWII), and the Chrysler dealer had his dealership converted into a six lane bowling alley. Today's kids (and parents) would have a tough time believing this, but Gene and I were at work every day but Sunday from 9:00 am till midnight, and often later on weekends. That's 90 hours per week or more. There were no machines; we did it all – lifting the ball to the rail, returning it, and resetting the pins. My weekly earnings were typically ten to twelve dollars, minus Social Security and taxes. And we walked home after midnight unescorted from downtown, about a mile or two.

Our main customers were soldiers from the Army Air Corps base eleven miles away, where the B17 Flying Fortress (a la the Memphis Belle) pilots and crews were trained. Our town had three movie theaters and no bars, so the soldiers bowled. There was a café up front, and I can still hear Tommy Dorsey's "Boogie Woogie" playing about every third selection on the juke box. It is still my favorite tune to play on a tape or CD. (I haven't caught on to iPods yet.)

Shortly before we went to work for the bowling alley, Gene and I had seen the movie "Harmon of Michigan." It was a true story about the 1940 Heisman Trophy winner, Tommy Harmon, tailback "Old 98" from the University of Michigan, and he played himself. Well, there was a soldier who frequently came to bowl with us, and he was the spitting image of the man in the movie. The other thing noticeable about him was that when he came, some pin boy was going to get hit with a pin. I think I probably had him as a customer more often than the others. That really didn't matter, because the boy in the next lane was as likely to get hit as the one in his lane. Both of us would bring our legs and feet up on the bench, turn sideways and shield our heads as best we could.

After more than 70 years I recently went on the Web and did a Google search for Tom Harmon. Guess what! He flew fighters *and B17s* in the war and earned a silver star and a purple heart. I know I can't prove it, but I'd bet a week's pin boy wages that our friend was the real Tom Harmon. There are way too many coincidences to not be real: the twin brother look, the strength of his arm, the branch of service, the equipment he flew, and the timing. So, Special Agent Gibbs of NCIS fame (aka Mark Harmon), if you're reading this, you could make a big fan of yours and your father's very happy by confirming or denying my supposition.

While I was working at the bowling alley, Mother had taken a Women's Ordnance Worker (WOW) job as a quality control inspector at the Army Ammunitions Plant in Milan, about 40 miles away. You've heard of Rosie the Riveter? She was the poster child of the WOW girls. Depending on Mother's shift, she would leave at ten and get home at ten, am or pm. We saw each other on Sundays. She later became the kitchen manager at the café in the bowling alley.

In January of 1945 we moved to Memphis, where Aunt Louise and Uncle Ervin were doing well with a mercantile company, and had arranged for them to hire Mother. They even bought a house that we would live in. The job required a car, so Mother bought a 1938 Plymouth, which would be the car I'd later learn to drive in. Still later, at age 19, I would buy my first car, a 15 year old 1936 Chevy Roadster convertible, with a rumble seat. My sister Jo's husband, James Lowery, the best body and fender man around, had bought it as a wreck and restored it to like new condition. I paid him $250 for it in 1951. My next car was a 15 year old 1940 Oldsmobile black sedan, that James said looked like something John Dillinger might have driven. My sister Bobbie's husband, JW Davis, put me on to that one for $125 in 1955. To this day I have never owned a car that ran as quiet and smooth as that one did.

Anyway, before long I was finally in Memphis Technical High School in the tenth grade,. At 5 ft. no inches tall, there was one student that was smaller than I was. Marilyn Hughes, arguably the prettiest girl at Tech, was 4 ft. 11 inches tall. I grew three inches the first year and was still the smallest boy there the next year.

Army ROTC was mandatory for all boys for two years. My uniform was a seamstress's nightmare. The pants had an 8 inch hem; the back pockets merged as one; the shirt sleeves had six inches tucked in, and the bottom half of the shirt pockets disappeared below my waist. One fellow enjoyed calling me half-pockets. The first day of my junior year, I walked into the music classroom and Bill Dickey called out "Hercules." It was like calling a 300 pound man Tiny. The next day Jim McMaster shortened it to Herky, and that was my name for the rest of my school days.

In my first year I bought a snare drum and signed up for the ROTC band, without ever having held a drumstick in my hand. The first day on the marching field, the director told me, "If you're going to make a mistake with that thing, make it loud so I can correct it." It is advice that I have given my students in computer classes for the last 30 years. By my senior year I was playing first chair drummer.

In my senior year I took an elective third year of ROTC, and was promoted to captain. There were two very good reasons for going that extra year. I wanted to be an officer so that I might raise enough courage to ask Marilyn Hughes to be my sponsor. She would wear a white uniform, march with the company, and attend the social functions with me. I did finally get up the courage to ask her, and she accepted and actually seemed pleased. The second reason I took another year was so that I would have a uniform to wear to school three days a week without having to buy it. My wardrobe was pretty much blue jeans and tee shirts (the white ones, like Special Agent Gibbs wears *under* his shirt).

After I graduated in June of 1949, Walker enrolled the next fall. The first day of registration he was in the hall when Captain Kirschner, the head of the ROTC program, stopped him and asked him for his name. When he told him his name the Captain said "I thought so. You're Johnny's brother. What instrument do you play?" When Walker told him he didn't play an instrument, he came back with "You'd better learn one. You're in the band." That day Walker came home and said, "Johnny, show me how to hold a pair of drumsticks." Until a very few years ago, Walker was still playing, with Gene Jernigan's (Dyersburg friend) 17 piece orchestra and with a small Dixieland combo that he, Gene, Bob Osburn and a few others had put together back in the 60s.

During the last week of high school, a bunch of us joined the Naval Air Reserves, and attended an eight week modified boot camp at the Naval Air Station in Millington, just 18 miles out of town. After the "Summer Cruise," as the Navy called it, I went to weekend drills once a month, and was on active duty two weeks in the summer. I was assigned to a squadron of TBM Avengers, the same kind of torpedo bomber that George H. W. Bush had been shot out of. Bush's plane was named TBF – same plane, different manufacturer. I had volunteered to be a combat air crewman, either turret gunner or radioman, they didn't specify which, but it never came about.

In the fall I enrolled in Memphis State College, but dropped out in November and went to work for the Quaker Oats Company's chemical plant as an office messenger, which involved maintaining the Purchasing Agent's inventory files, managing the mail room and running errands. I drove a company car home at night, so I could pick up the mail on my way to work in the mornings. I loved the job and all the people there. Then in June of 1950, the Korean "conflict" began.

A few days later I got a phone call from a close friend from high school, Edgar Buffaloe, my boxing mentor. He was turning 19 and worried about the draft, and asked how he could get into my squadron so we could serve together as our choice. So he signed up, and the personnel officer told him they had no opening in my squadron, but he would put him in VF791, the fighter squadron, and move him later. Hah! Before he got his uniforms and sea bag issued, that squadron got orders to active duty. The Navy needed those F4U Corsairs, fighter planes, right now. Within a few days they were in San Diego and training for combat aboard the USS Boxer. Wasn't that a fitting name for his ship? I've never told Edgar this, but it was probably Jim McMaster who got the last spot in my squadron. Jim's serial number was 333-6917 and Edgar's was 333-6918.

It seems the TBM torpedo bombers were outdated, so in November of 1950 three of us (just 3) from our squadron were issued individual orders. On Wednesday, January 10, 1951 I reported for duty, and was sent to the Naval Air Station at Jacksonville, Florida. The other two were assigned right there at NAS Memphis.

On Monday the 15th, I boarded a train for the 24 hour ride to Jacksonville with five others who had been called back to duty. They taught me how to play penny ante five card stud poker, and I made $2.95, enough to call my girl-friend after we got settled in. When we reached the station Thursday morning, it was about ten o'clock and we were hungry. We found the café in the station and took seats at the counter. There were six of us, one Rebel and five real live Yankees, from Wisconsin, Michigan, Pennsylvania, New York and Illinois. When one of them asked if we were too late for breakfast, the waitress said "Yes sir, I'm sorry, but we're all out of grits." They all looked at me, and one said "Hey, Ridge Runner, what the heck are grits?" I said "I have no idea. What's a ridge runner?" I had never seen a bowl of grits, and my home was maybe 200 miles from the nearest ridge.

Upon reporting for duty I was put to work at the Naval Air Technical Training Center, (NATTC), assembling lockers in barracks that had not been used since WWII. After that I was assigned to the Disbursing Office as a messenger, which means I sat around most of the day with nothing to do. I developed an affinity for the new Friden electro-mechanical desk calculators they were using to calculate the payroll, etc., and pitched in to give me something to do.

I never flew in a Navy plane again, except once as a hitchhiker for a weekend hop home to Memphis. So I changed my rate from aviation to disbursing clerk and spent the next two years paying the troops. I also never set foot aboard a Navy ship. When Jim McMaster heard about my getting individual orders, and the squadron staying on the ground, he quit the Naval Reserve and joined the Marine Corps. He returned home with a bronze star and two purple hearts.

After a year in Jacksonville I was transferred to NAS Memphis where I served my last year and was released to inactive duty on Friday January 9, 1953. I had already enrolled at Memphis State College (now University of Memphis), and classes had begun four days earlier. Thanks to the leading chief petty officer, with whom I didn't enjoy the best of relationships, I didn't get out of there as early as I would have if my immediate chief had been running things. Anyway, I rushed home to change clothes and catch a bus to the campus for what classes I could make that day.

Unfortunately, when I got home there was nobody there and I had no key. So I did the natural thing; I crawled through a window, changed out of my uniform and high-tailed it to MSC.

I learned later that the lady next door, who had seen me come and go in that uniform for a full year, called the police to report that a sailor was breaking into her neighbors' house. I was gone before they got there.

3
My College Days

College was fun. With the $110 I received every month from the GI Bill, and the money I earned in part time jobs, I was able to handle the $45 per semester tuition fairly well. I was actually solvent. I carried a morning paper route (on foot, paper on the porch, behind the door on rainy days, collect in person every Thursday and Friday and Saturday, and all that) from that January until the summer began.

Then I took ten days off in June to take a trip with a high school friend, Bob White, who had just graduated from Memphis State and was due to report to the Army. We stepped out on the highway with any part of Mexico as a destination, and with very little money, and with our thumbs out. The second car to come by stopped. Leon Drewry was our age and was on his way to a Mississippi town 138 miles south, but we wound up that night in San Antonio, Texas, about 750 miles away. Leon's brother was in the Air Force there, and he arranged for us to sleep over in a barracks. The next day we toured Nuevo Laredo, Mexico, then headed back up to San Antonio, where Leon left us after 1,380 miles of his original 138 mile plan.

Our next stop was Austin, Texas where we took a self-directed tour of the University of Texas campus. We found our way to the student bookstore and bought a couple of t-shirts with the big orange name of TEXAS on the front, thinking that might make it easier to catch a ride out of there. Sure enough, we caught one right away with a baseball fan who had a dozen questions about how the team was going to do in the next season. You would have thought Bob knew the coach, the way he made up answers without hesitation. That skill must have served him well later as a lawyer.

Entering Waco, we stopped and had a visit with another friend we had graduated from high school with, Don Isom. Don had joined the Air Force a week before I reported to the Navy, in 1951. In those days Don, Bob, another school friend, and I called each other Red, for reasons that won't make any sense, and really aren't worth telling. Bob and I still use that name when we get together, usually around Christmas time in Memphis. Anyway, the next time I saw Don was when Don "Figaro" Colvin and I drove back to Waco a year later for his (Don Isom's) wedding to Bobbye. I had the honor of being his best man. I talked to both of them yesterday on his birthday. The wedding must have been done properly, because it's lasted 60 years and still counting.

The next day we made it to Dallas and spent the night in a hotel. The next morning we headed up toward Tulsa, Oklahoma, still wearing the helpful Texas t-shirts. We wound up in St. Louis, Missouri, where we stopped in a barber shop to get a shoe shine, of all things. The crowd in there had a good time giving us a little ribbing about Texas. Bob was sitting up high in the shine chair, puffing on a cigar. The shoe shine man said "I hear they got chickens in Texas big as elephants. Is that so?" Bob casually thumped the ashes off his cigar and muttered, "The chickens are big enough to eat the elephants." That was the end of the Texas wisecracks. We finally made it back to Memphis after 10 days, in time for Bob to report to the Army, and for me to look for a summer job.

The rest of the 1953 summer I drove a truck (don't laugh) for Tiny Tot Tidiers, a diaper service company. Of course, this was long before disposables were available. The deodorant pills in the back of that van were the size of hockey pucks. At one house, as I brought out the wrapped package of clean diapers in exchange for a lady's laundry bag of used ones, she said that she sure was glad she didn't have my job. I told her I'd much rather have my job than to have hers.

The following summer, 1954, I went with two Sigma Phi Epsilon fraternity brothers, Walter Robbins and Gene Weaver, to Los Angeles and worked on the assembly line at the Ford Motor Company in Long Beach. Walter had a relative by marriage who was the plant manager, and he put us to work. I moved around, filling in for whoever was on vacation. Walter spent the summer driving the cars off the end of the assembly line.

While I was in Los Angeles my brother, Walker, was playing drums in a country and western band every other Saturday at a night spot in Memphis called the Eagle's Nest. On the other Saturdays a local boy Walker's age that dressed funny, wore a ducktail haircut, and had an odd name that rhymed with pelvis, was playing and singing and wiggling all over the stage with his shirt unbuttoned down to his waist. Thus entered the era of Elvis Presley.

When I returned to Memphis at the end of the summer the entire musical scene had changed from big band (real) music to rock and roll, and it has not been the same since. Walker's high school class of 1952 adapted well to the change; my class of 1949 never did. The Korean war had ended, we were returning to college or work, and we were not through with our music of Glenn Miller, Tommy and Jimmy Dorsey, Artie Shaw, Gene Krupa, Harry James, Benny Goodman, the Mills Brothers, Nat King Cole and other genuine musicians.

A brief singing career

Every spring the Delta Zeta sorority would hold their annual Follies, featuring competitive skits among fraternities and sororities, and Individual talents. In the spring of 1955 four of us from the Sig Ep fraternity organized a barbershop quartet. We called ourselves the Sing Eps. Wally Miller sang tenor, Larry Hilbun was our baritone, Jim McMaster, who gave me the name “Herky” and with whom I had sung in a barbershop quartet in high school, sang bass. I sang lead, the part that usually carries the melody, because I could no longer hit high notes and didn’t have a good enough ear to sing baritone. We learned one song for the Follies, “Ragtime Cowboy Joe,” and rehearsed it well enough to win the individual trophy. We earned a modest amount of money performing in the coming year, but more important, we got invited to a lot of parties and community functions.

Leon Nall had a combo consisting of him on piano, my brother Walker on drums, Ernie Skillern on bass, and Tommy Cogburn on guitar. Naturally, they picked up on our name and called themselves the Swing Eps. Then when Raymond Holmes got his rock and roll group together, they became the Rock Eps. Oh yeah - our fraternity chorus also won the All Sing competition three years in a row with Wally directing. The first year we had 32 pairs of lips moving, and sounds coming from 18 pairs of them.

During that same spring semester, I tried out for a spot on the cheerleading squad and was selected. After I graduated in 1956 Walker made the squad and was partnered with my former partner, Betty Jean Lauderdale. Who says college ain't any fun!!

Now for the running part

Actually, it's not entirely true that I didn't run while I was in school. In the spring of my sophomore year, 1954, Don Colvin (whom we called Figaro), told the guys in the fraternity I was fast, so they entered me in the 50 yard dash in the intramural May Day competition. I was told the speed merchant to watch out for was a fellow named Jerry Baldridge. As I recall, we ran it on grass. I don't remember who won, but I did beat Jerry by a foot.

The following year I was entered in the 100 yard dash and the 4x100 yard relay. This time we would be using the cinder track, and the track coach was the starter. Of course we wouldn't be using track shoes or starting blocks, just tennis shoes. In the South, we were not accustomed to the word sneakers yet; all such shoes were called tennis shoes. I was in one of the later preliminary heats, and I noticed that a lot of the guys were slipping on their starts, and not getting good traction. Naturally, I reasoned that if I got good traction I might get out ahead of some folks. So --- off came the shoes and socks. Sure enough, I got a good enough start and won my heat. There was a small break in the skin on the ball of one foot, so a Band-Aid was applied and I was ready for the 4x100 yard relay preliminaries.

Frank Land would start off, transfer the baton to Lynwood Bargery, then it would go to Larry Hilbun, and finally to me for the finish. So we walked to our stations on the track to wait for the race to begin. We were in lane one. Now remember, this was Memphis, Tennessee. It was May. The temperature was not in the upper 90s yet, but it was hot. By the time Coach Allen fired that pistol and Larry got the stick to me, I felt like I had been standing on the top of my mother's wood burning cook stove. And I was a few steps behind Bubba Leonard, the quarterback of the football team, in lane two. I thought I made up a little of the gap, but came in second behind him. We'd get 'em in the finals, I felt sure.

Since this was not something I had trained for to any great extent, I was pooped and flaked out in the grass to catch my breath. Some of the guys came over to check on me, and one of them said, "Look at your feet!" Have you ever seen a kid's shoe that had lost all the stitches from the front of the sole, and the sole was hanging down from the tip to almost the middle of the shoe? That was what my feet looked like. The entire ball of each foot was hanging down like peeling wallpaper. Under where the skin used to be it looked like raw sausage, with tiny bits of cinders ground into it.

Somebody quickly fetched two paramedics who were standing by with an ambulance. After a good look at my feet, their response was "Sorry, we can't do anything for you." Great. And they were gone!

By this time half of the student body had gathered around to see what this fool had done to himself. And in that group of rubberneckers was the graduate student trainer for the football team, "Snake Doctor" Williams. The man took over like a field general, or at least a drill sergeant. Four friends were directed to carry me to the team locker room. No, it didn't require four men to carry my 136 pound frame across the football field, but I soon learned why he wanted four. Two of them carried me and deposited me on a table, on my back. Then each man took his post. Larry Hilbun was on my right shoulder and arm, Leon Nall was on my left, and Minor Holland and a fellow named Thornton had a leg each. With what would come next, Snake Doctor knew it would take all four of them to keep me still.

Step 1: He took the scissors to each of those sheets of loose (live) skin and removed them.

Step 2: He poured, not dabbed, not swabbed, but poured alcohol on the ground-up sausage-like balls of my feet. After he finished cleaning out the cinders and doing whatever else he did, he told me to lie there until I could get the strength to get up and make it to the shower, clean them up and he would bandage them. By the clock, it was 15 minutes before I could sit up, much less hobble to the shower.

I still don't know Snake Doctor's real name, or whether he ever practiced medicine or not, but the doctor who later changed my bandages was an amateur pre-med student compared to Mr. Williams.

But May Day was not over yet.

You see, I had been taking a folk and social dance class to be near a girl I had been dating, Bobbie Nell Conlee. For the festivities on stage in the college auditorium that night, we were to do a featured polka dance as a couple. You know, where you spend a lot of time on the *balls of your feet*. And a lot of it involves *bouncing backward* on said balls of your feet. No way, Jose.

Well, it turned out that Bobbie Nell was not ready to scratch the act. "Isn't there some way? Please." I thought, maybe we can get Bob Trantham to do it, if he can learn the routines this afternoon. He's a good dancer, agile (captain of the cheerleaders), a fraternity brother, and a good friend. He gave it a sincere try, and then he just as sincerely gave it up. That means I've got to do it, and I can't even walk!

Just before the curtain opened on our show, two fellows carried me to center stage where I leaned on Bobbie Nell's shoulders to take some of the pressure off my feet. When the curtains opened, I was all smiles, bouncing around the stage, and having a good time. Only once, when I took a bounce step backward, did I make one huge grimace, but covered it rather well (I thought). When the curtain closed, the guys rushed back onstage and lifted me off her shoulders and carried me off. The act was saved. Bobbie Nell was saved. The dance class instructor was saved. I was a hero in my own mind. I was on crutches for two weeks.

And I got a lousy "B" in Folk and Social Dancing.

The Interview

In my senior year, 1956, a few of us were sitting around talking about what comes next, and one fellow asked me what I was going to do with my math degree. I was to graduate in August after the summer semester. I had changed majors three or four times and still had no clue what was in store for me. But there was one thing of which I was certain. I was not going to teach school. Then somebody suggested that I try the IBM Corporation, because they had a great reputation, had businesses all over the globe, and hired a lot of mathematicians and engineers. That sounded like a good idea, so I'd think about it.

Apparently that conversation had opened my reticular activating system, because a few days later I noticed an ad in the *Memphis Commercial Appeal*, looking for engineers and mathematicians to work in Kingston, New York, where IBM was developing computers for the US Air Force's air defense system, known as SAGE. SAGE stood for Semi-Automatic Ground Environment. When American Airlines, along with IBM, later developed the first airline reservation system, they borrowed from that name and theirs became known as Semi-Automatic Business Reservation Environment. You may know it as SABRE.

So I made the phone call, and met with their man in downtown Memphis on March 17, 1956. In addition to the usual questions about my grades, jobs, and extra-curricular activities he asked if I knew anything about IBM equipment. I told him I was working for a truck line at night, using an IBM billing typewriter. Then came the $64 question: "Do you know anything about computers?" I didn't even know they had started making them yet, so I told him all I knew in this one sentence. "I remember in a freshman math class, Dr. Kaltenborn said they *would be* using a number system that consisted only of ones and zeroes, but I don't remember what he called it." That vast amount of insight earned me a plane ticket to New York for a second interview. That turned out to be the only job interview I had or even asked for before I graduated.

After I had spent a full day of interviews and touring the IBM plant in Kingston, I returned to school and told my friends that I had been offered a job with IBM as a mathematical programmer. When asked what that meant, my reply was that I had no clue, but they told me they'd teach me.

I sent back my acceptance of their offer, and immediately received a letter telling me that from that date until reporting date I would be paid a signing bonus amounting to 50% of my proposed salary for that period. I liked the corporate world already.

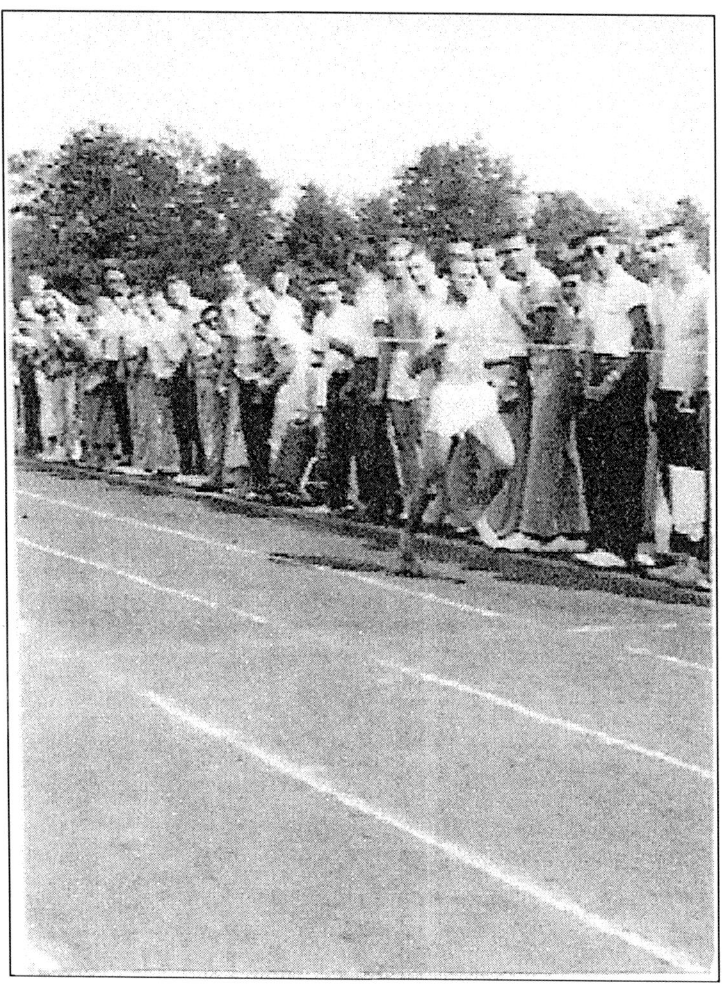

You've heard the expression "burning up the track?" This cinder track got even; it burned up my bare feet, in the May Day events at Memphis State College in 1955.

4
The IBM Years

School for me was over on Friday, August 17, 1956, and I was to report to work in Kingston, New York on Monday, August 27. After parties on Friday and Saturday nights, Alvin Iverson, a Sig Ep brother and fellow cheerleader, and I left on Monday in my 1956 Ford for points east. We stopped in Nashville and bummed a cot and a couch off of Bob and Wilda White. He was out of the Army, married, and in law school at Vanderbilt University. The next night we spent at the YMCA in Roanoke, Virginia. You see, I had spent most of the bonus money on the car, dark suits, white shirts, "sincere" ties and the mandatory hat. The room at the YMCA was so cold we got up about 4 am and continued on to Philadelphia, where we spent the night at Ivan's uncle's house. I left him there and pulled into Kingston on Thursday.

Kingston was a very interesting town. It's about 100 miles up the turnpike north from New York City. The population was about 28,000 people, and the IBM plant accounted for 6,000 more. Besides designing and building the computers for SAGE, the Air Force air defense system, there were 65 programmers writing maintenance programs to keep them operating efficiently. Also, they trained engineers who would service them. The engineers were there for nine months at a time, and received per diem allowances. That accounted for apartment ads in the paper that read "IBM only," and signs in the window of a clothing store that read "Sale – IBM white shirts." When I asked a man at a service station how to get to the IBM plant, he told me to get in my car Monday morning and follow the white shirts.

The people in Kingston could spot an IBMer a mile off, even over the phone. I called a dentist's office to ask for an appointment, and was told "If you can wait until next Tuesday the 6th, election day, it's your holiday and we can see you then." On another occasion I called the Firestone store and asked the price of a set of tires for my car. The man gave me the price and said that they could come out to the plant and put them on there. Neither of them had bothered to ask if I worked for IBM.

I reported to work on Monday August 27, 1956. Right away they asked me for my motel and restaurant receipts and automobile mileage for the expense account. What? Motels? Restaurants? Mileage? Expense account? For a guy who was almost 25 years old, had worked in the corporate world a short while and served in the military, I guess I was still a country bumpkin. This expense account idea was one more thing I liked about the corporate world.

The next thing they told me was to not unpack just yet. I would be going to Boston over the weekend for seven weeks of programming school at an MIT satellite.

Back in the classroom

Boston was great. IBM put me in a very nice motel in Bedford for which they paid $6.00 a night (back home a Holiday Inn was $4.00 a night). I got laundry and dry cleaning allowance, $7.00 a day for meals, and six cents a mile for my car expenses. I was living high on the hog.

Our instructor, Gene Pulk, was a former MIT math professor, and he was really good. Our product was the AN/FSQ-7 computer, the largest computer ever built, designed for the SAGE air defense system. You've read stories about computers that took up a whole room. This one took up a four story building, 40 of which were to be located around the planet to keep track of things in the air and determine which things should be there and maybe which ones should not. The building had one door, no windows, and enough air conditioning to cool a small town. When I visited one later, I asked why the buildings were not placed underground. The answer was "If it works, it doesn't need to be underground. If it doesn't work, then it doesn't matter."

The computer covered more than 8,000 square feet of floor space, had 58,500 vacuum tubes, 1,500 miles of wires, 120 display screens, rows of magnetic tape drives, rows of magnetic drums (we didn't have magnetic disks yet), and weighed 275 tons. That's over half a million pounds. Oh yeah, it also had a "huge" memory of 8,192 bytes (they were 33 bits and we called them words). My job was to write programs that would predict which of the vacuum tubes that controlled the memory units were about to fail. And I didn't know an electron from a spark plug.

I had never learned to study, and I thought this might be a good time to start. Seated next to me in the programming class was Rex Depew, a former math professor from Florence State College in Florence, Alabama. That happened to be where my Aunt Muriel worked in the registration office. My competitive spirit got the best of me, and I had to do well to compete with Rex. On every quiz or test that we took, Rex and I made identical scores. If I missed two questions, Rex would miss two, but not the same ones. This silent competition continued, known only to me, until the last week, when we had a case study to do. Rex was missing. When I asked Gene what happened to Rex, he told me that he had already completed the full course earlier, and this was a repeat refresher so he could begin teaching it the next time around. Wow! I almost felt like I'd been had, but actually I felt good about that.

What happened next made me feel even better. I learned that in all IBM training classes, and there were jillions of them, they rank the students at the end of the course. It turned out that I wound up in second place of the 33 students. As a result of that, and my instructor Gene's phone conversations with my manager-to-be, whom I hadn't met yet, I had a 7.14% increase in pay before I got back to Kingston. I not only learned how to study, I learned *why* I should study. (Actually, my idea of studying was to pay very close attention in class. Truth is, five of us played penny ante poker in my room every night after class, until just before the ice cream parlor closed. I had a banana bucket every night; that's a banana split on steroids. I must have been born with perfect metabolism, because the 14 pounds I put on in those seven weeks leveled off in no time. That was the last time my weight ever fluctuated more than five or ten pounds.)

So I became a programmer for the largest computer ever built.

That winter it snowed 28 times in Kingston. The temperature dropped to 25 degrees below zero, and this was before we had a wind chill factor to tell us how cold it really felt; it was actual temperature. Eskimos are built for that environment, but this Southern boy was not. So on November 8, 1957 my favorite company and I parted ways. One of my friends predicted to me, “Reb, I bet you’ll be married within a year.” You know what! I did get married one day shy of a year later on November 7, 1958 to Gwen Ford, a girl I had a crush on in high school, but never had the courage to ask her out. She was recently divorced from Alex McCollum, a friend from junior high and high school, and had a six year old son named David, whom I raised and was proud to call my son.

After a year or so back in Memphis, I realized that the job I was in was going nowhere. As usual, a new door was opened for me. I ran into a fraternity brother in the Toddle House diner, and learned that he had an appointment for an interview with IBM. Gwen and I were encouraged by the thought that they might need people locally, so I went to see them. An appointment was given me, and I spent half a day taking aptitude tests.

The District Manager’s approval was necessary for the branch office to rehire a former employee, so his assistant flew into Memphis to interview me. The IBM custom was to lock the door when someone leaves (they probably thought that anybody that would leave was mentally deranged). But computers were about to become practical commercially, and I had three things going for me. I had programming experience, my personnel record stated they were sorry to see me go, and according to him I aced all the aptitude tests they gave me. So with the District Manager’s approval, on May 4, 1959 I went back to work for IBM in the Memphis branch office as a Systems Engineer Trainee, and restarted my career in the computer world. I felt much more comfortable about supporting my new family with my favorite company.

On September 1, 1959 John Hurd Jr. was born. Don Isom's wife, Bobbye, was there to help me pace the floor. Don was out of the Air Force and out of college, and we were neighbors. Don was having interviews with IBM, which led to his moving to Kingston, New York, working in the same department I had been in.

Then in January of 1963 I was transferred and promoted to Instruction Manager of the District Education Center in Kansas City, Missouri where we trained customers and new sales and systems engineer employees. Two other highly significant events occurred in Kansas City that year: Kevin Hurd was born on April 11, and the Dallas Texans NFL football team moved to Kansas City and became the Kansas City Chiefs. Kevin is still their number one fan.

Moving away from the South, there were a few language customs that were different than in other parts of the country. In the South we were taught as young children to respect our parents and other adults, especially those in authority, such as teachers, and to address them as "sir" or "ma'am." Well, when young John Jr. was in about the third grade he had a lady teacher from Boston. And everybody knows that up there they not only have their own language customs, in many ways they have their own language. So when John would respond to a question from his teacher, he would say "Yes, ma'am," or "No, ma'am." Each time he did that she would "correct" him with "John, that is not necessary. A simple yes or no is all you need to say." John would then remind her that that was the way he was taught at home to show respect for elders. One day he came home from school and said that she was still telling him to stop using the term ma'am. I told him not to let it upset him, and that if she continued I would meet with her and ask her politely to respect our wishes. So the next time she corrected him, he told her that his daddy said that if she did that again he would come to this school and have a talk with her. So far as I know, she never "corrected" him again.

We made our home in a new subdivision in Overland Park, Kansas. It was a great place to live, and a wonderful neighborhood. Everybody on Eby Street was from some other place, the men were all 31 years old and made $10,000 a year, none of the wives worked outside of the home, each family had 2.4 kids, we had lots of house parties, and two annual 12-man Eby Street golf tournaments. I was a terrible golfer, but I had a lot of fun.

While we were living there, the boys were about 14, 7 and 3 when David got the notion to call his biological father (Gwen's ex-husband), Alex, and invite him and his new wife and their two sons to come and spend a few days with us. Alex accepted, and a date was set. And *then David decided to tell Gwen and me.* On the Sunday afternoon when they were expected to drive up, every couple on Eby Street was sitting on their front porches waiting to see if it really happened!

Well, it did really happen, and we had a ball. I had a great time introducing Alex and David around the area as "My son David and his father, Alex," or "Alex McCollum and our son, David."

After two years in the Education Center and then a year as Systems Engineering Manager in the Kansas City Branch

Office, I made it to the district office in Shawnee Mission, Kansas, where I became a special representative for the Votomatic – the punch card voting system. So if you think you know what went on in the ill-famed presidential election in south Florida in November, 2000, you probably don't. Most of what you know is probably what the folks in the media told you that night, and most of that was wrong. So sit tight, fasten your seat belt, and relax. You are about to hear...

5
The Rest of the Punch Card Story

IBM had a product called the Porta Punch. It was a system that could be used to place a pre-scored punch card into a portable device and punch holes with a special stylus. It was used for such things as taking inventory in a warehouse, by punching information such as part numbers, bin numbers, shelf numbers and quantity on hand. Dr. Joseph P. Harris took this idea, and developed a device that could hold a ballot printed on pages that could be turned to expose a row of a card which had these same pre-scored punch positions that would line up with a candidate's name or an issue to be voted on.

I won't go into the details of the innards, except to say this: The card was to be inserted into the device (not a machine), and the pre-scored rectangular chips were to be removed with a special stylus that was attached by a chain, so it was always there in the voting booth. The card could only be inserted one way. When inserted properly and punched with the provided stylus, a clean removal of the chip (chad) occurred every time. If the card was simply laid alongside the ballot pages in an attempt to line up the numbers on the card with the numbers beside the ballot choices, and/or use something like a ballpoint pen instead of the stylus, a dimpled or hanging chad would be the result every time. This only happened when the voter was super smart, knew everything, and refused to pause a few seconds to follow the simple directions given by the poll worker.

Before a new voting system could be sold and used in a given state, enabling legislation had to be passed, with very strict rules about the use of the system. For example, a few days before an election was held with the Votomatic system, there would be a public test announced and scheduled to confirm that the computer in use was properly programmed to tally votes for that particular ballot, with all of its variations by precinct, and a complete application of that state's unique rules for tallying. And believe me, some states had their own unique rules of tallying. There will be more on that later.

After the public demonstration, the program and the sample ballots that were tallied were sealed in a vault by the election officials. On election night, after the polls were closed, the program was removed from the vault, the seal broken, and the same certification procedure was repeated. After the tallying of the day's votes was concluded, the program was again sealed and locked safely away, along with all the ballots.

My responsibility in all of this was everything but manufacturing and selling the devices and the cards. I wrote programs, conducted the training classes for precinct workers, conducted the tests, and "presided" over the entire operation on election night, and did the same for the occasional recount that occurred. Later, I had a territory as a salesman, and still later became the plant manager for the ballot card production.

Now let's get back to Dr. Harris, the inventor of the whole thing. He had sold a few counties and municipalities, including Braintree, Massachusetts and the three counties, Fulton, DeKalb and Cobb that make up Atlanta, Georgia, and a few other locations. IBM bought the system from Dr. Harris and retained him as a consultant.

Our first on the job training that I participated in was a student government election on the campus of Louisiana State University (LSU). It was 1966, and as I remember, it was in February. I wrote the program that ran on LSU's IBM 1401 computer, and we had 22 representatives present to assist, and mostly to learn, including my District Manager Larry Myrick, and a couple of division executives. It went off well, and I learned a lot from it.

My next election was the real thing, in Waukegan, Illinois for Lake County. It was Flag Day June 14, 1966. I wrote most of the program on an airplane from the west coast to Chicago, so the name of the program was AA, for the airline I was on.

This is where I learned about the many different procedures the various states might have in the way they elect folks. I don't know if they still do it this way, but in the race for Representative in the General Assembly there were three to be elected in each district. That meant that each voter had three votes to cast. In the general election there would be two candidates from each party, and the voter could vote a straight party choice for the entire ballot or select the candidates individually, or use a combination of both, which would override the straight party vote for that office. If a straight party vote was made, then the two candidates from that party would each receive one and a half votes. But if candidates were selected individually, regardless of a straight party vote, then selecting one candidate from either party would give that candidate three votes, or selecting two would give each a vote and a half, or selecting three would give each candidate one vote. Simple, huh?

If I had a way of proving it, I would bet the ranch that there had never been an accurate tally for that office in any election where paper ballots were used. When we installed the system in Sangamon County, which includes the state capital Springfield, they used paper ballots for the absentee voters. In 127 precincts, the number of absentee ballots ranged from none to 11. Not one precinct had tallied the ballots correctly. Many of them did not even add up to a multiple of three votes. This is in no way intended to criticize the people who tallied the votes. I read the instructions that were given to them, and if that had been my only directions I'm not sure I could have done any better.

The election went off without a hitch, and I think the experience with the paper absentee ballots pointed out how much more accurate their new system was than the old way.

My first recount

One of my early elections was in Rockford, Illinois, in the county of Winnebago. The night of the public certification of the software accuracy, I learned a couple of things: (1) Not to put up with negative time wasters and (2) To choose my words carefully when being interviewed by the media.

One of the local officials warned me that the chairman of one of the political parties would probably give me a bad time. Sure enough, as I was preparing for the evening's events the chairman approached me, introduced himself, and said he had some questions for me. I said fine, ask them. Then he added "I have to tell you first that I don't believe in IBM." I responded with "Then there's no point in my answering your questions, if you won't believe me anyway. Excuse me, I have work to do." And I never heard the questions.

After the test was completed and everyone was satisfied with the results, a newspaper reporter arrived late and asked if I would go through the test again for him. As I was doing so, he asked me what would happen if I wrote the wrong instructions. I reminded him that this public display was to assure everyone that I had tested it many times already to be certain that every vote would be properly and accurately counted. Somehow, I managed to say that the computer wouldn't know if I was right or not. I said that it was a supersonic moron that does only what the program code directs it to do. When I got back to the IBM District Office in Shawnee Mission, Kansas, Larry Myrick, my District Manager, asked me "What kind of interviews do you give?" He had a Rockford newspaper, as did IBM headquarters, with the front page headline "Moron Proves Perfect in Election Test." The story was positive, but I took the word moron out of my professional vocabulary.

A few nights before the election I learned one more thing, having nothing to do with elections: "When in Rome, do as Romans do, speak Italian." I was joined in Rockford by two fellow IBMers: Jack Gerbel, who had sold the system to Winnebago County, and Arthur Murray, another special rep whom I loved to page in hotel lobbies and airports. We asked one of the ladies in the elections office for a good place to get dinner. She said that in the Italian ward, there is an excellent Italian restaurant named Maria's. Great, we'll go there.

Maria's Italian Restaurant had maybe 20 people on their wait list. As Art and Jack approached the hostess's stand to get our name on the wait list, one of them said to the hostess "You must be Maria." At that same time I spotted a short authoritative looking woman approaching and I said aloud in my best Italian accent, "No no. Quella non e Maria. Ecco e Maria qui." (Translation: "No, that is not Maria. This is Maria here.") The lady walked straight up to me and asked how many were in my party. I answered three, and she said "Come with me." True story. I wasn't even sure if I had the words in the right order, but it worked. And the food was indeed great.

OK, I'm getting to the recount. In Ward Five, that same Italian ward, Mr. Gaziano beat Mr. Sparacino in a local office race by 24 votes. I went to Larry Myrick, my District Manager and the following dialog took place:

Me: Why don't you go with me? It'll be a good learning experience for both of us.

Larry: No way.

Me: Why not?

Larry: What if you go up there and some guy with slick black hair and garlic breath asks you if you want to see your wife and kids again if this vote doesn't come out his way?

Me: You've been watching too much television.

Larry: I'm not going.

And he didn't.

Now, I know Larry had other priorities, and I actually saw no need for his going, but I enjoyed the conversation anyway.

Well, they counted every one of those votes by hand and then counted them again by computer, and Mr. Sparacino still lost by the same 24 votes each time.

For the record, in my 15 years in the voting business, nobody ever suggested to me that it would be worth my while to see that a vote came out a certain way.

My second recount

This one was a doozie. It was the general election in Will County (Joliet), Illinois in November 1968. Remember the unique way of tallying I described for the office of State Representative in Illinois, where every district elects three people? Well, the man who finished fourth was *ONE* (1) vote shy of being elected. Just one. Have you ever thought that your one vote didn't amount to much? You should have been around for this one.

When I arrived in Joliet, I counseled with the County Clerk, and suggested that we have someone punch several sample ballots as we did at the public certification ceremony and then count them to verify again the accuracy of the software. Then we would let the loser choose 5% of the voted ballots, as the law permitted, and count them by computer. If the results came out the same way, it's game over. She agreed, and the rest was up to me.

When I walked into the hall that night with about 50 people present, you could have cut the tension in the air with a knife.

It was as if half of them hated me and the other half were looking out at the parking lot hoping to see my white horse.

On the way over there, little Johnny Hurd, who usually goes out of his way to avoid confrontations, had stepped into a phone booth and put his "take charge" face on. I knew that I had to be 100% in charge and on target, otherwise it could be a long night. I took the floor and announced the plan, and the loser's attorney immediately challenged me. He argued that it would take hundreds of sample ballots and we would never know if we covered all the possible combinations. I told him it would take exactly 64 cards. I explained that there were six punch positions that affected this race: the two straight party positions and four more for the candidates. With 64 cards we could punch every possible combination of those six holes, including all 6 positions punched, and a card with no punches at all.

"So in your professional opinion, it would only take 64 cards to cover all combinations affecting this race," said he. Said I, "No sir, that is not an opinion. It is a mathematical fact." Obviously irritated he said, "Would you list all those combinations?" I asked for a pad and pen and listed all 64 of them in binary sequence, and handed him the pad and pen. He then asked if I would sign it. I took back the pad and pen, signed it, and proceeded to punch 63 cards and throw in one blank one.

We counted the sample ballots, they picked the precincts they wanted counted, we counted them, and I left for home. And guess what? The dude was still one vote shy.

I conducted several other recounts over the years. Not one result was ever overturned.

In 1969 IBM divested itself of the voting system. They did not like publicity of any kind, good or bad. In the company's history since 1914, they had never even spent a dime on advertising. So when the voting system represented one tenth of one percent of the revenue and 72% of the publicity, they dropped it. Jack Gerbel and the team in the San Francisco area left the company and bought the whole thing from IBM, including the services of Dr. Harris. I was moved to Regional Headquarters in Washington, D.C. to help work us out of a job. After a year there they began to talk about White Plains, New York, and in June of 1970 I bailed out and headed south to warmer climate.

In a short while Jack Gerbel called me from Chicago, saying since he was in the neighborhood (600 miles between Chicago and Memphis was "in the neighborhood"), he wanted to drop by and say hi. OK. Turns out he wanted me to fly out to Berkeley, California and talk about joining the team at Computer Election Systems (CES), which I did. So from that time until April of 1980 I covered the states of Tennessee, Mississippi, Georgia and both of the Carolinas as an area sales manager.

In May of 1978 Gwen and I went our separate ways (peacefully), and remained the best of friends. In June, 1980 I got married to Sandy Stone, originally from Hopkinsville, Kentucky. Her father was the town doctor there for 45 years, and delivered his only child, Sandra, on January 1st, 1947 at 12:01 AM, making her probably the first baby boomer born in the Central time zone. The girl born at that hour in the Eastern zone became the poster child with all kinds of gifts, etc. When I met Sandy she had boxes full of trophies and ribbons for swimming, diving and baton twirling from her high school days. She had also won the title "Miss Kentucky of Baton Twirling." In her college days at Ole Miss she was one of the Rebelettes, and was feature twirler at the Sugar Bowl game when Archie Manning (Payton's and Eli's dad) was the quarterback there.

After our honeymoon in the Bahamas, Sandy and I made our home in Dallas, Texas, where I had relocated in April as manager of the ballot card production plant in Addison, a suburb. In December of that same year Sandy's father died, on the same day that another famous Kentuckian, Colonel Harland Sanders of KFC fame, did. Her mother had been diagnosed with cancer, and Kevin had come to live with us for his last year of high school. Life was a bit of a struggle, with everyone in different places, but our spiritual training kept us going.

Meanwhile, Computer Election Systems (CES) had been sold to a holding company and 63 employees had been terminated, including the president. One of the new owners, Tom Wiley, appointed himself president.

In May of 1981 on a Wednesday I got a call from the new president, setting new plans for my future. We had sold Cuyahoga County, Ohio (Cleveland) a system and also Cook County, Illinois (Chicago) was a new customer. The president wanted me to move to Cleveland *this weekend* and help prepare for the primary election in September, then move to Chicago in time for the general election in November. What? Move to Cleveland in three days and in four months move to Chicago for good? Well, he said I could just get an apartment and commute for four months. Gotcha, Tom. Ain't gonna happen, mate.

The next morning after I left for work, Sandy said to God, "If you've got something else for John, tell him today!" Later that morning I had another call, from Peter Evans, a close friend I had worked with in the early years of voting with IBM. I had neither seen nor talked to Peter in about ten years. The complete verbatim conversation went like this:

Marilyn:	John, it's for you.
Me:	John Hurd.
Voice:	What are you gonna do for lunch?
Me:	I'm gonna eat it.
Voice:	What time are you going?
Me:	When you get here.
Voice:	I can be there in 25 minutes.
Me:	I'll be ready.

On Saturday I met Burk Muldoon, the owner of the company Peter was working for. He had an involved system for managing business forms, running on a mini-computer, which were fairly new and PCs hadn't quite hit the scene yet. (What we now call a hard drive was called a Winchester, because the spec sheet resembled those of a Winchester rifle.) His programmer had left him with 73 programs, none of which worked completely, and he needed a good programmer now. Of course I had never heard of Burk's computer manufacturer, much less the programming language, but what the heck. What else is new?

The next Monday I called our vice president, Tom Barnes, one of the survivors at CES headquarters, and told him I would go to Cleveland for two weeks, then he would be on his own. They made other plans, and that was my swan song with the voting business.

After a couple of years of putting Mr. Muldoon's software in good shape, Peter and I left his employ and took a stab at selling home computers. Then in early 1984 Kevin was attending the University of Tennessee in Knoxville, and Sandy and I moved back to Memphis. My brother Walker was head of a computer department (I had recommended him in 1962) at State Technical Institute at Memphis, a two year college staffed by instructors from the industries they represented. He kept urging me to come to work there as an instructor, so on July 1, 1984 I did just that.

I had barely had time to find my way around the campus, when Professor Bob Osburn finally persuaded the president and the board to let him set up a Microcomputer Resource Center to provide the training and resources the area would need when PCs started flying off the shelves. As soon as he got the approval, Bob came to me and asked if I would be his assistant, and I said sure. I had known Bob in junior high school, and again when he was an IBM customer. He was a data processing manager at Schering Plough when they were installing an IBM 1401 tape and disk system, and that was my last assignment as systems engineer before my promotion to the Kansas City Education Center. Four years after opening the Mid-South Microcomputer Resource Center at State Tech Bob returned to the IT Department and left me as Director of the Center for the next 12 years, retiring June 30, 2000.

South Florida, November 2000

Then along came the presidential election in November, 2000, with all of the hoopla about hanging chads, dimpled chads, disenfranchised voters and so on in the counties of Dade, Broward and Palm Beach, which included Miami, Fort Lauderdale and Palm Beach. I was not there, but I still have the scars on my feet where Sandy nailed them to the floor to keep me off the next southbound airplane.

There were more untruths and misleading statements put forth that night than I had heard from my TV since I could remember. I had been part of the team from Computer Election Systems that put the systems in Dade and Broward Counties (Miami and Ft. Lauderdale) about 25 years before, and to my knowledge they had done pretty well with it. Why else would they have kept it that long?

At 7:00 pm Eastern time that election night, one of the major TV cable networks announced that the polls were closed in Florida and they were projecting Al Gore to be the winner of the state, meaning that he had won the presidency of the country. I heard it estimated that upon hearing that report approximately 10,000 Republican Florida voters went home and did not bother to go to the polls in the Central time zone, which is heavily Republican, and begins 160 miles east of the western edge of the state.

Was that announcement about all of the Florida precincts being closed merely an "oops" – an oversight? If you believe that, as many people do, then you apparently are not aware of the truckloads of money the TV and radio networks and the print media spend in preparation for a presidential election.

They have very elaborate databases that they use to determine not only which states are key to the election, but also which precincts to place workers and volunteers in to report from often during the day, to give them the pre-tally information to make such predictions. It is a highly sophisticated and competitive race to be the first to call a winner and be correct. They cannot afford to leave anything to chance. This had been going on for at least 40 years, since primitive computers were on the scene, and the time zones have not changed during that time. Do you really believe they had forgotten that Florida is divided into two time zones?

I have no first-hand knowledge of why they picked the three specific counties (the third being Palm Beach County) to challenge the votes, but I suspect that, because of the heavy concentration of voters that favored their party, their "recount legal team" and telemarketing organization were stationed there quite some time before the election.

Remember the so-called "butterfly ballot" they displayed on election night to show how the voters might have been confused? When you have a long list of names in one race, such as presidential electors, they must all be visible at the same time on the ballot pages. I have designed many such ballots without a problem, and had to admit that that one, as it was shown on the news channels, seemed a little unclear to me for some reason. They displayed it again on the second night, and I felt the same way. Then on the third night James Baker of the other party showed one that was clear as it could be. I met the Supervisor of Elections from Palm Beach County later, and she confirmed my suspicion, that on the first and second nights they used copies, which were obviously not camera-ready. That did not matter; the public had already been convinced that it was a confusing ballot.

There is one thing I did know with 100% certainty, without having to be there. It was stated over and over again that night and for two weeks after that "More than 17,000 voters in Palm Beach County alone were disenfranchised; their ballots wound up in 'Spoiled Ballots' envelopes, and their votes were not counted." All of that was true except for the words "disenfranchised" and "not counted." In any election in all of the 15 states I have worked in, the rules are the same. If you are issued a ballot, and change your mind or make a mistake, you may return your ballot, receive a new one and vote properly. You have up to three chances to get it right, whatever the reason. Since every ballot has to be accounted for, the ballots that are returned are placed into a special envelope marked "Spoiled Ballots." I actually heard a commentator on one of the TV cable channels, a full two weeks after the election, repeat the disenfranchised charge. He caught himself and said, "Well they weren't really disenfranchised, but it doesn't matter now." Are you kidding me???

I will add three other personal observations about that election:

(1) The Supreme Court did not elect George W. Bush President of the United States. They called a cease to the circus that had more recounts than "Jaws" and "Rocky" had sequels.

(2) If Al Gore had carried my home state of Tennessee, which *he represented* as a United States Senator, it would not have mattered one whit what the state of Florida had done.

(3) Whether you liked Bush or not, he won the election playing by the rules.

6
Sprinter's Glossary

I know placing a glossary in the middle of a book, instead of in the back, is not the conventional way of doing things, but to enjoy the rest of the book I thought it necessary that you understand the language of the sport. For example: when people learn that I'm a runner, their first question is usually "How far do you run?" or "How many miles do you run in a day?" To the first question, my answer might be "About a block." I'm told the average city block is about $1/8^{th}$ of a mile, which is 220 yards, so I wasn't being a smart aleck, just having fun. To the second question, the answer is "I don't run miles; I'm a sprinter." In either case, I usually have to explain myself. After the explanation, the next question is almost always "When is your next marathon?"

Here, then, are the translations.

NSGA – National Senior Games Association, the organization that puts on the Olympic style games for men and women who are fifty years old or older by the end of the year in which they first compete. The games include most track and field summer games, and several others such as golf, tennis, swimming, three-on-three basketball, softball, etc. Competition is divided into five-year age groups: 50-54, 55-59, and so on. National competitions are held every two years in the odd numbered years. Qualifying events for the national games are held by the individual states in the previous (even numbered) year. Most states require qualification at one of several local venues held throughout the year, in order to compete for the state games held later that year. States and local districts hold events every year, but only the even numbered years are qualifying years for the national games in the following year.

Some states invite athletes from outside their states to enter their games, but some do not. If a person earns a medal in a state other than his/her home state, it does not take away the medal from the residents who finish first, second or third within their state. e.g. Sam Smivitz, from Wyoming, competes in Mississippi's games and wins a gold medal. Sam gets his medal, but Roscoe Splivens was the best of the Mississippi contestants, so he also gets a gold medal. If it is a qualifying year, each of them qualifies for the Nationals in the next year. For those who do not place in the top three or four to qualify for the nationals, there is a qualifying time that can be met to qualify, no matter where they placed in competition. Some athletes will go to a neighboring state to qualify, if they were not able to do so in their own state for any reason or even if they did.

Senior Olympics – The National Senior Games Association (NSGA) and most of the states refer to their Senior Games as The Senior Olympics.

Meter – One meter is 39.37 inches. In Jesse Owens's days (and in my college days of the fifties) track and field events were measured in yards, feet and inches. Somewhere along the way they were changed to the metric system.

Kilometer – One thousand meters or 62.137% (almost 5/8) of a mile.

100 Meter Dash - 109 yards and one foot, or 328 feet, and replaced the 100 yard dash.

200 Meter Dash - 218 yards and two feet, and replaced the 220 yard dash.

400 Meter Dash - one lap around the track, lacks eight feet being a quarter of a mile in lane one and replaced the 440 yard dash, which was a quarter of a mile. In the old days you could run four laps in the first (inside) lane and that was a mile. Some people who are not familiar with these figures think they have jogged a mile when they haven't. Depending on how long the straightaways are and how tight the curves are in a given track layout, each lane out is approximately 22 feet longer around than the one to its left. That is why, when running the 200 meter or 400 meter dash, the starting point for each outside lane is moved up a distance to compensate for that. That distance is referred to as the stagger.

800 Meter Run – Two laps around the track, and replaced the 880 yard (half mile) run.

1500 Meter Run – Three and three quarter laps around the track. It is sometimes called the metric mile, though it is actually 93.2% of a mile.

5K Run – Five thousand meters (5 kilometers), approximately 3.107 miles. Races longer than 1500 meters or one mile are usually run in the streets.

10K Run – Ten thousand meters (10 kilometers), approximately 6.214 miles.

Marathon – Approximately 26.2 miles.

Half Marathon – Just what the name implies, approximately 13.1 miles.

Runners and Joggers – The vast majority of runners fall into one of these categories. They usually have red muscle fiber (slow twitch), meaning the muscles receive more oxygen. They can replace oxygen as they use it. Most can carry on conversations as they run. Their events are timed in minutes, or even hours. Their form of running is considered an aerobic exercise. What, then, is the main difference between a runner and a jogger? According to *Runner's World* magazine, it's an entry form.

Sprinters – Athletes who run the very short races – 50 meters, 100 meters, and 200 meters. The 400 meter run is considered by some to be a sprint event (dash), especially college and Olympic athletes. These events are almost always held on an oval track. The sprinters wear very lightweight shoes with no support and from seven to ten spikes, usually 1/8 inch or ¼ inch long, on the forward soles of the shoes, never on the heels. Spikes are never referred to as cleats. Starting blocks are also used to give the sprinter a more explosive start off the beginning line.

Track shoes – See **Sprinters**, above.

Flats – What the rest of the world calls running shoes. They of course have no spikes, are heavier than track shoes, and offer more support. Runners and joggers wear them to run in the streets. Sprinters use them on the track during their warm-up routine. Most sprinters change into track shoes once they finish the warm-up exercises and stretches and begin their sprint practice or the actual scheduled races.

Electronic timers – The starter's pistol is linked to an electronically controlled digital timer, which is automatically activated by the firing of the pistol. The runners are automatically photographed at the finish line, and the distance between torsos is measured in thousandths of a second by ruler-like markers at the bottom of the picture. This is displayed on the screen of a computer.

Bib Number - The number, usually three or four digits long, that identifies each contestant in the games. It is on a rectangular cardboard tag that is pinned to the front of the runner's singlet (shirt).

Hip Number - When using electronic timers with a camera at the finish line, sprinters are usually issued an adhesive-backed tag with a single digit indicating the lane you are in, in that specific heat. It is adhered to your shorts on the side that will face the camera at the finish line, usually the left side.

PR - Personal Record. i.e. Your best recorded time for a particular event, usually in a specific age bracket.

All American Awards – There are pre-set standards that one must reach to achieve All American status. In running events, the times are set in hundredths of a second. There is a time requirement for each five-year age group for each running event. It has nothing to do with whether a reporter likes you, or your coach is a good lobbyist. You either made it or you did not. There are no gimmes and no arguing. As of this writing the author has achieved All American recognition in at least one of the 100, 200 and 400 meter events for 17 out of the past 18 years – 1997-2014. I missed it in 2005 for the 200 meter dash in the 70-74 age group by one hundredth (1/100) of a second. The requirement was 32.00 seconds and my time was 32.01. The next year I broke the Florida record for that event in the 75-79 age group by half a second. The previous record was 33.16 seconds and my time was 32.66.

World Class – Again, there are no subjective decisions involved. For each individual age there is a world record for each event. If your mark compares to that record with a 90% efficiency or better, you are considered, by *National Masters News,* to be World Class. There is no award for this achievement.

7
Gotta Love Those Volunteers

Most of the people who work at the meets are volunteers, and do it because they love the sport. Without them, there probably would not be any games. Most of the time they do an excellent job of seeing that things run smoothly. I always pause to thank the ones that I come in contact with, after my events are over.

We are all human, and we all might occasionally get things a little bit off. But none of the boo-boos I've seen were worth getting emotional over, and some were rather amusing.

Once I was competing as an outsider in another state, and my first event was the 50 meter dash. When the gun fired, one of the fellows had already taken a step or two out in front of everybody. I managed to pass him, and thought I had won the race. But the other guys wailed so loudly about his jumping the gun, the official brought everybody back to run it again. Now, wasn't that fair!?? I beat the jumper and everybody else in the heat. But since he fouled, instead of DQing him (disqualifying), he got another opportunity to beat me. I never said a word, because it meant nothing to me beyond the day, and I was a guest anyway. Oh yeah, I won the second time also.

On another occasion, I was competing in my first Tennessee Masters Championship. I finished the 100 meter dash in second place behind John Wall, with whom I later became good friends. When I went to the scorer's table to get my silver medal, the lady told me that I had won the gold. I assured her that John had won, despite the hand-held stopwatch that showed me with a better time. Then we ran the 200 meter dash, and the same thing happened again. John won the race, but the stopwatch again showed me with a better time. You see, they had a timekeeper for each lane, but nobody had the responsibility of watching to see who actually won. When the gun goes off 100 meters from the timekeeper, approximately three tenths of a second will pass before the sound of the gun reaches the finish line. So one timer starts the watch with the appearance of smoke from the gun barrel (properly) while the next one starts at the sound, and it's almost impossible for either to get it just right.

Sometimes you run too far; sometimes you don't run far enough.

It was the Tennessee Senior Games championships. We were running the 100 meter dash, and when I thought we should be through, we were still 10 meters from the finish line. It turned out that Harvey Foster was the only one who had noticed we had lined up at the 110 meter hurdles line, but nobody would hear him until after it was over. How did I know we had run too far? It's the OCD thing (I count things, including steps when I run). Besides just feeling like it was off, I knew I had taken too many steps for 100 meters. Now, they were in a pickle over how to record the times. I calmly explained to them that the only thing they could do would be to divide our times by 1.1. It took them over an hour to exhaust their other sources and conclude that I was right. I must have been the only person in the stadium with a math degree. Of course, it couldn't be exact, because we don't usually run the extra 10 meters at the same speed we ran the rest of it, but at least it was more accurate than what we had, and we still knew who won.

Then there was another state championship, at the same venue. In the 400 meter run, the man in lane eight came in elated, saying "I've never run 400 meters in that time before." I told him he still hadn't. They started them from the 800 meter starting lines, meaning everybody had twice the stagger (extra starting distance) they would normally have had. In other words, lane eight had about a 50 yard advantage, lane seven somewhat less, and so on down. The poor guy in lane one is the only one who actually ran the full 400 meters. I don't know if they did anything to correct that one.

In another local event, where one goes to qualify for the state finals, we were on a different track than usual. Somebody had measured the starting point for the 50 meter dash and indicated it with a wide blue tape. After my age bracket ran our heat, I approached the starter, Matthew Dobson, and told him that it was closer to 54.27 meters than 50. How did I know? Because it took me almost three extra steps to reach the finish line. I think what must have happened is that someone measured 50 *yards,* instead of meters, from the starting line to place the tape, which would mean that we started 14 feet early. Matt couldn't believe I actually counted the steps. (I think the shrinks call that a psychosis.) Matt is an excellent coordinator and starter, a marathoner, and a former amateur athlete of the year for the Pensacola Sports Association.

And sometimes it's not the volunteers

As of this writing I have lived in Florida more than eleven years. During that time I have competed in 67 races in and for the Pensacola area and the State of Florida. In those 67 events, I won 66 gold medals and one silver. The silver one came about this way.

Hurricanes Ivan, Dennis and Katrina had ruined the surface of the track where we usually held the qualifying events for the Pensacola area, so we borrowed a high school track which was pure asphalt. The 50 meter dash was the first race, and I was to be in the second heat. I was so preoccupied with having to run in flats on asphalt, that I didn't pay attention to the starter's rhythm, the number of commands, etc. Big Huge Mistake. Always pay attention to such details, especially on such a short event where you have no time to recover or catch up. I was expecting the usual "Runners to your marks," then "Get set," then the firing of the gun. I hadn't noticed that the man *didn't even have a gun*. So we lined up and I heard the starter say "Runners to your marks." He skipped the second command and the next sound I heard was a meek toot from a toy horn. I looked around and thought "What was that?" It was then that I noticed that all the others were running in the direction of the finish line, so I thought I'd better join them. By the time I caught up with Bob Martin, we were at the finish line. I wasn't sure who had won, because Bob had lunged so hard that he had skidded across the line and lay there with what seemed like half the skin peeled off his left arm. According to the stopwatches he took it by one hundredth (.01) of a second. My bad.

So what was my time?

We were in the national championships in Baton Rouge, Louisiana in 2001, and the preliminaries of the 100 meter dash. Don Beck (Maryland) and I were in adjacent lanes. Don got a lead on me, but I overtook him about 75 or 80 meters out. My time was 13.92 seconds, and Don's was 14.09. The scorekeeper had known that Don had the early lead but didn't notice that I had passed him. So he posted my time by his name and his time by mine. Maybe they hadn't told him about the purpose of the lane numbers on our hips. Anyway, Don was the one who came to me and told me they had recorded the times improperly. Since we both had qualified for the finals the next day, it shouldn't have mattered. What did matter, though, was that 13.92 was world class time, and 14.09 was not. That one never got corrected.

That was my last time to run that event in less than 14 seconds, so far as I know. I say that because the next day in the finals, Don did beat me 14.33 to 14.35. We'll never know what anybody's actual times were though, because of what happened just before that. On our first start, somebody jumped the gun and it was called back. Since the gun activates the clock, it had ticked off a good part of a second before the gun sounded again to signal the false start. The problem was that the volunteer college student at the scorekeeper's table failed to reset the clock after the false start. Don and I were both in the top six, but neither of us medaled, nor did I get recorded as having qualified as world class in that event.

Then came the national championships of 2013 in Cleveland, Ohio. It was the first time the 50 meter dash was included at the national level. In the preliminaries I had the best time, Ronald Gray was second, and my good friend John Wall from Tennessee was third. In the final heat I won again, Ron was second again for silver and John won the bronze. Since that was the first time the event was held in the national games, the winning time establishes a new record. Right? However (there's that word again), the clock did not activate at all, so I will hold that record until 2015, but the next man to claim it won't know whether he beat it or not.

I went to the referee and the person who maintains records and suggested they use our preliminary times, since we finished in the same order both times. Nope; they couldn't do that. I told you there were no gimmes in the Games.

Breaking News

Here's another "however" for you. I just today received the Results Book from the 2013 National Senior Games, and they did do just what I had asked them to do. They recorded our preliminary times again as also the final times. So the official record is 8.72 seconds, which happens to be world class time.

8
Why Do I Run?

What was it that made me, a young man of 60, decide to do something that I never got to do in high school or college, that most boys do when they are in school, and soon after forget it or maybe continue it through their college years, or even further? I could give you all the standard answers: (a) I want to improve my health, or (b) it's so refreshing to be outside and feel the wind in my hair, or (c) I really do need to lose some weight, or (d) I can join a running club and make some new friends.

While these are all really good benefits one might enjoy, the truth is: (a) I've been blessed with good health naturally for most of my life; (b) I've had very little or no hair since college days anyway; (c) my weight hadn't fluctuated more than five pounds in the previous 35 years, and (d) the kind of running one would do in a running club is counter-productive to the training a sprinter needs.

I think the real answer to why I started to run is that I wanted to see if I could get to be good enough to enjoy some of the fun things I didn't get to do while I was in school. If I trained really hard, I could envision myself perhaps someday winning a state championship. Well, if I had wanted to do it then, then why didn't I? The answer to that question is, because I was too little. When I was in the 10th grade in high school I was 5 feet 0 inches tall and weighed 92 pounds, about the size of a typical fifth grader.

In 1937 I lived in Dyersburg, a small town in Tennessee. School was starting in September, and I would turn six in October, the day after Mickey Mantle did. (No, I didn't know Mickey; I just thought I'd throw that in, that being the only thing we had in common.) I wound up having to ride a school bus to a school out in the county, while my best friend next door, Gene Jernigan, walked less than a mile to school in town. I never did understand that until my older sister Jo explained it to me a few years ago. The school officials would not believe that I was old enough. They came to our house and told my mother she had to be mistaken (lying) about my age. The birth certificate did nothing to change their minds, so I wound up spending the first grade in a different world where everyone was a total stranger to me. The next year the school I should have been in had no choice but to take me in. I had very good grades, and maybe that helped.

By the way, Gene didn't turn six until the next March. I didn't understand that either. That problem stayed with me all through high school. Five days before graduation I enlisted in the US Naval Air Reserve, with my mother's written permission, because I was just 17. The officer who inducted me and another kid didn't believe I was 17 years old. After we took the oath he looked at me and said, "That means you swear that you're 17." The boy next to me was just 16, but he was 6' 4" tall, so he didn't doubt him.

When you're the smallest kid around, there is one thing you can almost be sure of being included in: being picked on and shoved around. There is another side to it also. When there is a physical project to undertake, like building a kite or making a magazine rack in Vacation Bible School, some bigger boy will assume you're too little to do anything like that, and do it all for you. The down side of that is, that between the bigger helpful boys, my three older sisters, and losing my father at age three, I didn't learn much about being a handy man, much less about how to cook – traits I still don't have.

The external stimulus

It happened in the spring of 1992. We were attending a weekend seminar in the home of Peter Ragnar, the "Magic Man of Mystic Mountain" in east Tennessee. Peter related the inspirational story of an Olympic sprinter from another country, and the courage and persistence that were required to see him through all of the physical challenges he endured to finally win the Gold Medal that meant "Best in the World."

I don't recall the athlete's name, but on the way back home my name seemed to be changing to "Walter Mitty." That was the name of a movie about a man who lived in a world of day-dreams. (The Danny Kaye version. I do not watch remakes of good movies.) Anyway, I began to reflect on the years when I was too little and too underdeveloped to do any of the things that most kids either do or daydream about. I wondered "What if I were to start training and see if maybe, just maybe, I could beat some of the speed merchants of my earlier years? After all, they are all old men by now." I was to learn later that when you get to the national scene of the Senior Olympics, there may be as many as 12,000 athletes there that are fifty and over, and the old ones must be in some other sport, because they certainly did not seem to be on the track.

A few days after Peter told his story I spotted a neat story in the Memphis newspaper about a college friend of mine named Jim Mathis. (There's that reticular activating system again.) Jim was an outstanding 440 yard and 220 yard sprinter at Memphis State. He had been coaching high school track, basketball and softball all those years since school, and was competing in the Masters and Senior Games (aka Senior Olympics), and breaking state, national and world records in the 100, 200 and 400 meter sprints.

To my surprise they were still using starting blocks and wearing spikes, but with one big difference. The cinder tracks had given way to a rubberized surface, so the spikes were a good bit shorter. As Jim's son, Jay, commented in the newspaper article, the old spikes of Jim's college days could have been used to climb telephone poles.

Now, here is the encouraging part of that story. The competition was divided into 5-year age groups: 55-59, 60-64 etc. Jim was 57 and I was 60. I'm thinking that means I'll only have to line up next to Jim two years out of every five.

So the training began, pretty much in secret. I was not ready to listen to people laugh at me, or tell me I was being foolish, or to act my age, or I would ruin my knees, or any such nonsense. For the first year, very few people were aware of what I was doing.

My only experience with regularly scheduled running had been with the boxing team in high school, and later in the Navy. (I got out of standing a lot of midnight watches, got to wear dungarees to the evening meal, and got steak on the day of a fight.) We called it road work. After I gave up boxing I began to notice highway signs that read "End road work." I thought that was a pretty good idea, so I did just that. I ended road work.

In 1992 I began my training by walking, at which I had always been pretty good. After two or three months of vigorous walking, I wanted to see what I could do in a 40 yard dash. Using a 100 foot extension cord I measured off 40 yards (120 feet) on a street that had little or no traffic at 6 am, and took the four-point stance. Now remember, I had not run a step since this began, and my warm-up consisted of a little walking. The mental gun sounded in my head. I threw my right foot and left arm forward, and my right arm backward. Then the left foot went forward, and the right one again and then – POP – I thought it could be heard a block away. My right calf felt like it had been shot. That was July 13, 1992. I learned volumes that morning about warming up thoroughly and starting out light.

OK, so now I at least knew something I shouldn't do, but I had no idea what I should actually be doing. I searched the shelves at the major bookstores and all of the books seemed to be written for people who run miles and kilometers and weird things like that. People like that have clubs they can join and run with their buddies and learn from each other.

I had known forever that I was not a distance runner. I was the kid who didn't smoke or drink, but still couldn't run more than a city block without being winded. I had learned about white muscle fiber and red muscle fiber in 7th grade science class. But all I learned (or remembered) was that red muscles received more oxygen. I did not learn that they were called slow twitch and fast twitch muscles. I did not learn that a person with red muscle fiber (slow twitch) could replace oxygen as he used it, and so could run farther and longer before becoming winded. People with white fiber (fast twitch) were more capable of bursts of high intensity activity lasting several seconds, but had to rest to recover. So, armed with this ignorance, I had spent 60 years believing that I was somehow physically different from normal people. Maybe I had small lungs, or a weak heart, or something like that. After all, I did have pneumonia when I was six years old.

Anyway, if I aspired to be a sprinter I had better learn how to do it. So I browsed the book stores again to see what they had to offer. There seemed to be a plethora of books and magazines on running, but they were all about 5 Ks, 10 Ks and marathons. But in my reading I came across an ad for Carl Lewis's training video, *Sprinting*, with Carl and his coach from the University of Houston, Lou Tellez. Carl and I had one thing in common: each of us ran 39 steps in about ten seconds. The difference was that by that time Carl had finished the 100 meter distance, and I had almost 30 meters more to run.

From the newspaper article about Jim Mathis I got the contact information for the Tennessee SportsFest, held every summer for everybody from little boys and girls up to the really old. It wouldn't be until next June, so the training continued. I called their office in Nashville, and asked about previous results in my age group. I had to know what I'd be up against. Then I went to my doctor for my annual physical checkup, and confided in him about my ambitions. I had been training for a month and had dropped 10 pounds. He was pleased, but told me I had a hernia that needed attention. Ouch. All right, let's get this over with; I have a track meet in six months. But the surgeon he sent me to said, "Nope. You have a loose ring, but no hernia." Hooray!

June 12, 1993 finally came, and I entered the 100 meter competition in my first meet. I was pleasantly surprised at the welcoming attitudes of the other athletes. The first man we met there was Hugh Powers, who would be one of my opponents. It was a Memphis day in June, and Hugh was very gracious in inviting my wife, Sandy, to sit with his group and enjoy the shade of their huge umbrella. What I was not impressed with was the way the whole thing was organized. We were supposed to run in the early morning, but did not go until almost two o'clock in the afternoon. There were only two others in my age group, Hugh and Ed Redditt. Ed won, and I managed to beat Hugh for second place. Sandy was really excited, because I received a 2nd place ribbon.

Two weeks later we went to Nashville for the state finals, and it was the same dis-organization, only worse. Instead of running at one o'clock, we ran after four o'clock in the afternoon. None of us had even had lunch, and I missed getting a bronze medal by about a foot. It was Bob Alexander, Ed Redditt, Carl Vaughn and then me. But I felt great, and The Games had begun for me.

Meanwhile, there was a retirement party going on back in Memphis for my former boss at State Tech, Bob Osburn. They said that Walker had looked around the crowd and asked "Where's Johnny?" When they told him where I was, it was complete news to him. Sandy and I did get there in time to enjoy most of the party.

Then a few days later the laughing, that I had wanted to avoid, began. A friend asked me how I had done at the state finals. When I told him I finished in fourth place, he said “Heh heh. How many did you beat?” Then the “toot your own horn” attitude, which I had also wanted to avoid, began. I answered “Including you, probably about 200,000.” That was the last time I was aware of anyone poking fun at my new hobby.

By the next May, 1994, I had discovered the Senior Games, and entered the local events to qualify for the state. I also discovered that even though Jim Mathis was only 59, he was in the 60-64 age bracket because of his age at the end of the calendar year. I finished in second place for the silver medal, but I only got a brief glimpse of Jim as he left the starting blocks.

For the rest of the summer of 1994 I accumulated three silvers (including my first silver at the state level) and three bronzes at the local and state levels, competing primarily with Jim Mathis and Bob Alexander from Memphis, and John Wall from Cookeville, Tennessee.

By the fall it was time to spread my wings. So Ed Redditt, the man who had beat me in my very first meet, and I went to Hot Springs, Arkansas on October 1st. Their state finals were being held, and outsiders were invited. This also attracted two ringers from Oklahoma, Glen Stone and Bob Santine. Ed managed to hold his own with them, but I wound up in fourth place in the 50m, 100m and 200m, just a breath or two ahead of Sid Montecino from the New Orleans area and a few others, but out of the money.

After the three events were over, the others were getting ready to leave for home, but there was still one race on the schedule that I had never trained for and the others were not interested in – the 400 meter run. With but a few exceptions, most good sprinters do not run the 100m, 200m and 400m, but Glen and Bob were lingering around with Sandy and me while I contemplated the thought of going home empty handed. I had no idea if I could even run 400 meters, much less sprint it. Glen advised me to not try to sprint it, just run four pretty good 100s back to back. Their words and body language seemed to be trying to very politely tell me to be smart and go home. As I glanced over at Sandy, she did a "lip read" message that said "Go for it." That was all I needed, so I put my spikes back on and headed for my blocks.

I followed Glen's advice, and ran what felt like four 100 meter strides at just better than a pretty good warm-up pace. Coming out of the last curve with 100 meters to go I was maybe ten meters behind Jimmy Culp. My first thought was to try to out-sprint him to the finish line. My second thought was if I did that and stiffened up, I might get nothing but winded, because I had never trained for the 400m at all. So I told myself to hold on to what I had and maybe I could take a piece of silver home. I took the second option, and made the trip home with a silver medal, feeling a little better about myself.

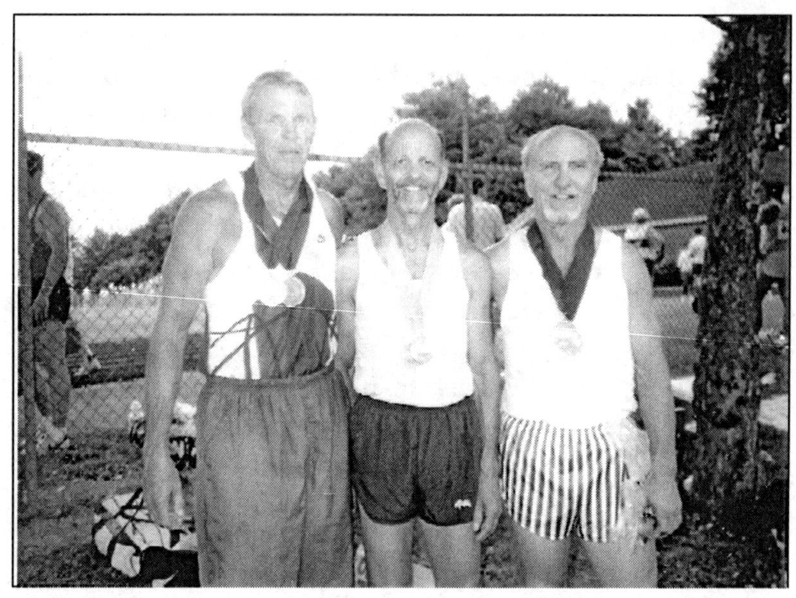

Left to right: Jim Mathis, John Hurd, Bob Alexander at Tennessee Games SportsFest in Chattanooga, TN June 1994. They are wearing gold medals; mine were bronze. Jim and Bob were my early supporters and competitors upon my entering The Games.

9
1995 – Time to Go to the Nationals

I knew I was probably not ready for prime time, but patience is not a real virtue of mine. I had to see what the national scene was like. I remember when I told some IBM friends that I was going to buy a set of golf clubs, back in 1962. The advice I received was don't keep score for the first year. That may be good advice for normal people (Sandy insists I was not born on Planet Earth), but it's wasted on a compulsive score keeper. How are you going to know if you're improving if you don't keep score? I had to know where I stood and where to go from here.

So I mailed in my entry form for the National Senior Games in San Antonio, Texas, and in May of 1995 headed southwest. I entered the 400m, the 200m and the 100m, so naturally my bib number was 421.

In my age bracket, 60-64, there were 62 men entered in the 100 meter dash, so it was necessary to have preliminaries, semi-finals then finals. The same was true of the 200m and 400m, where the headcounts were 43 and 39. In the 100m I made it to the semi-finals, but placed 18th in that one, so did not get to the finals. It was the same story in the 200m, where I finished 15th in the semis. In the 400m, there were 24 slots to fill in the semis, and I had the 23rd best time in the prelims, but based on times and finishing place in the heats, I was not one of the 24.

I was not overly impressed with my numbers in San Antonio, but I knew three things I was going to accomplish in the next national event in 1997. First, I was going to drop the 400m. For a beginner, that was just too much, to train for all three of them. Second, I was going to finish in the top six of one event or the other, because at that time they only gave ribbons for fourth through sixth place. Third, I was going to make All American in at least one event.

Meanwhile, between San Antonio and the Tennessee state finals in July I sprained an ankle, so I entered only the 100m, and got my first gold medal at the state level.

That September I went back to Hot Springs for the Arkansas games. I won the 50 meters in 7.00 seconds, world class time. In the 100m event Lowell Bonifield and I tied, but he out leaned me, so he won. As we lined up for the 200m, I asked him to not do that again, because it was too stressful. Wouldn't you know it; he leaned into another tie. But this time they said my whole torso was over the line, so I got the gold. Now I was a champion in two states!

On to the 1997 Nationals

Just before it was time to leave for the 1997 games, Bob Alexander dropped by my office at State Tech for some reason. As I introduced him around, my staff could not believe I was going to drive 1,425 miles to Tucson, Arizona to run with this man for six races (two events including prelims, semis and finals) that barely lasted a total of two minutes. "Why don't you just do it here? Seriously, John, you can fly to Phoenix FREE and rent a car for the short drive to Tucson," they said. (John Jr. was with Piedmont Airlines, which later became US Air, US Airways, and now American Airlines, all as a result of mergers.) My argument was that I couldn't get my starting blocks on the plane, and I wanted my own car there. The truth was that I actually enjoy driving cross country, and after more than 3,000 flights during the 15 years while I was counting ballots I was simply tired of flying. So in May I took off in my 1987 Honda Accord hatchback, with my two goals in mind that I had set two years earlier. I wanted a ribbon (4th through 6th place) and an All American certificate. The All American standard for the 100m dash for ages 65-69 was 13.80 seconds, and for the 200m it was 29.50.

On May 24, 1997 the National Games began. In the 100 meter prelims, I was second behind Joe Summerlin with 14.34 seconds, good enough to run again in the semi-finals. I improved to 14.14 in the semis, but still behind Joe and Bill Melville in that heat. I did make it to the finals, though, where I ran 14.18 and finished eighth out of nine places. Being the eighth best in the country should have excited me. After all, it was ten places up from where I was the first time, in San Antonio. But there was no ribbon and no All American certificate.

The next day was the 200 meter prelims. I thought I was doing fairly well in lane 2, but coming out of the curve I heard footsteps in lane 1. It was Halbert Goolsby, a good friend that I graduated from high school with, passing me. I had forgotten that he had a good finishing kick. I finished second with 29.71 behind his 29.65.

The following day was the 200m semi-finals. I improved to 28.83 seconds, 0.67 seconds better than the All American target, and was third in the heat behind Jim Stookey and Bill Melville. We still had one more to go – the finals.

In the finals the next day, coming out of the curve I counted four bodies ahead of me. I said to myself, that's all you get; no more. At the finish line it was Jim Stookey, Harry Brown, Bill Melville, Joe Summerlin and Johnny Hurd at 29.16 seconds, followed by a tie for sixth and Halbert Goolsby in eighth place at 29.71. I had a fifth place ribbon and an All American certificate. The moral of this story – If you don't have a written goal with a date on it, you're probably just having a good time.

When I got back to work at State Tech, my Dean, Carol Luce asked me how I did. When I told her I placed fifth in the nation, she exclaimed "That must be in the top 1% of something." I had worked too hard to put up with approximate math, so I helped her out a bit. "Carol," I said, "There are maybe 33 million people in this country age 65 or older. We know that at least four of them can outrun me for 218 yards and 2 feet." Sorry, I couldn't help that one.

Two months later in the Tennessee finals I won the 100m, followed by Bob Alexander, then John Wall and four more. Then in the 200m I got the gold again and Bob and John swapped places for second and third. In the 400m, George Barry got the gold, Bob the silver, and I got the bronze. Oh yeah, I also made All American in the 200m again.

In the 1998 Tennessee games it was Ed Redditt, me and John Wall for the top three in the 100m and 200m. Ed was still beating me, but I was getting closer and still making All American in the 200m.

In November of that year the *Memphis Commercial Appeal* ran a nice story about me with a picture, and my crew at the Computer Resource Center of State Tech cut it out and posted it on our bulletin board. That turned out to be another one of Commander Spock's "random factors" that operated in my favor. A short while after that, one of my Lotus 1-2-3 students, Paul "Sam" Pearson, read the story and asked if he could meet me at the track some time and work out with me. You bet, I said. Any time.

Sam was 29 years my junior, and a former sprinter/hurdler at Louisiana Tech. Remember Terry Bradshaw, who won four Super Bowl rings as Pittsburgh's quarterback? He was a Louisiana Tech product also. They do produce some great athletes. Anyway, Sam showed up as scheduled, and we trained together from February 1999 till June when he moved to Fayetteville, Arkansas. Sam was much more than just a friend to work out with; he was the only "trainer" I've had in my 21 year hobby.

Sam was not a paid, hard charging driver, but he did keep me honest. Every step that I ran, Sam was in the next lane to my right, just ahead of me. He could hear my footsteps and know what kind of effort I was putting out. At the end of a sprint Sam would say, "Tell me about your run." At first my answer would be something like "Gasp. I'll get back to you." Pretty soon, though, I was able to answer him in real time. I realize now that he was teaching me to focus. Every now and then Sam would say, "Let's rock and roll." Even today, when I'm ready to go for my week's goal, I might say to myself, "Let's rock and roll, Sam."

My two best training sessions came during that four month period with Sam. On May 1st we ran a 100m, then it was time to rock and roll with a 200m. I ran a 28.70 and used up all my gas (or so I thought). No way. We rested 10 minutes then did another 100m, and I clocked in at 13.41. But we still had a 300m and another 100m to do before we practiced starts with the starting blocks.

For that time in my brief career, each of those was a really good time for the practice field, but to put them back to back in the same workout was something I was not accustomed to. But now I knew what my goals would be for the nationals in October in Orlando, Florida.

Several days later I had a similar session. Want to hear the goofy part of this story? On each of these training sessions, the meals on the days before were identical: Blackened chicken sandwich, fries and Diet Pepsi for lunch at Back Yard Burgers, and for dinner I had pepperoni pizza and Diet Coke at Ci Ci's Pizza Parlor. Go figure.

Later in May we had the Memphis games to qualify for the state, and I finally beat Ed Redditt in the 100m. I think he had a sore foot. By July Sam had moved to Arkansas. At the Tennessee finals I scored a hat trick, winning the 100m in 14.14, the 400m in 69.00, and the 200m in 29.16. In the 100m and 200m John Wall was right behind me, and in the 400m I beat George Barry by two seconds. To be honest, I think George was about half sick, but he would not admit it. That was the only time I ever beat George. And I made All American in both the 200m and the 400m.

10
1999 – Disney Sports Complex, Orlando, FL

Several youngsters have moved up into our age group this year, including Bill Wright and Dennis Melanson from Massachusetts, Andrew Branch from New York, Ernest Walls from Ohio, Robert Reid from Virginia, Sydney Tate from Idaho, and Anthony Morrone from Pennsylvania. There will be 36 contestants in the 100m, and 44 in the 200m. There will be no semi-finals for either event; from the preliminaries, nine men with the best times will qualify for the finals. The schedule is: Thursday, October 21st (my 68th birthday) 100m prelims; Friday 200m prelims; Saturday 100m finals and 200m finals.

My goals are: 13.80 in the 100m (13.80 is All American), and 28.70 in the 200m (29.50 is All American).

I managed to pull off a win in the 100m prelims with a 13.80, on the nose of All American, 0.07 seconds ahead of Anthony Morrone. It was my PR (Personal Record) for that event, but I'm still not sure whether it counts as All American, since it did not happen in the finals. So to be certain, I'll have to do it again on Saturday.

The next day in the 200m prelims, I was in second place rounding the curve, but pulled out ahead and won it with a 28.50, another PR and it exceeded my goal for that event. At the curve I could see John Wall waving and yelling for me, and after the finish I got a big bear hug from him. Again, that's what it's all about.

Now it's Saturday, time for all the marbles. I don't have medals in mind; I'm running against the clock.

The 100m final turned out to be the closest crowd at the finish line I had been a part of. The new kids had a field day. Wright (age 65) and Branch (66) tied at 12.86 for 1st, Stookey (69) was 3rd at 13.28, Walls (65) 4th at 13.31, Reid (65) 5th at 13.33, Summerlin (67) 6th at 13.37, Melanson (65) 7th at 13.38, Hurd (68) 8th at 13.47 (another PR and All American) and Harold Oliver (67) 9th at 13.90. The *National Masters News* called it the most competitive event of the Games, pointing out that all eight of the top winners recorded World Class times.

Later the same day we had the 200m finals. This time we had still another youngster show up – Paul Johnson (65) from Texas, who smoked everybody with a blistering 26.29. The rest of the field was 2nd Wright, 3rd Branch, 4th Walls, 5th Summerlin, 6th Stookey, 7th Hurd at 28.60, 8th Tate and 9th Morrone. This was not my best showing in placement, but according to the clock it was, hands down, my most successful to date.

Thanks, Sam Pearson.

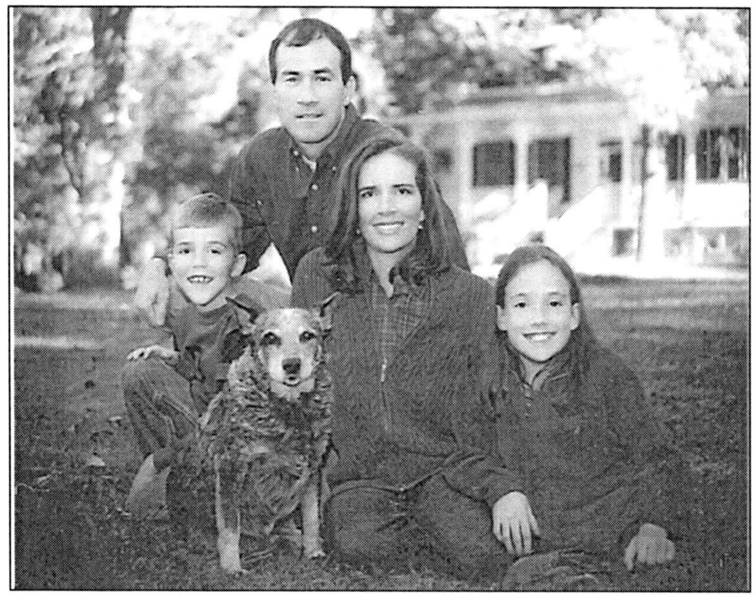

Left to right: The Pearsons, Paul, Sam, Donna and Bailey. The only personal trainer I've had. Sam just adopted me for a few months before moving to Arkansas.

11
They're Watching You

No, I don't mean the government, though that may be true too. I mean, when you take up a sport in a competitive capacity, sooner or later you're going to attract some attention. It may come from your family, friends, neighbors, co-workers, the coaches where you train, the athletes that train there, the soccer moms and football moms that bring their kids there, and their kids, and certainly your competitors. Maybe even the media. All of them can become good friends, especially your competitors.

For 21 years, except for the short time I spent with Sam Pearson, I've been training pretty much by myself. I remember that for the first few years I would go to a competitive event and watch the "big boys" to see how they did their warm-ups, how early before the first event they began, what kind of pre-game stretches they did, etc. After a while, I began to feel like some of them might be watching me for the same reason. So I guess it's natural.

New acquaintances

Speaking of Sam Pearson, he's a good example of what I mean. He just happened to be in a seminar at the time when my story was on the bulletin board, and I just happened to be teaching the seminar he was in, and a good friendship developed from that. We still hear from him every Christmas with pictures of him and Donna and the kids, Bailey and Paul. After moving to Arkansas, Sam got back into running again in those races that have K's in their names.

When I said that I trained alone most of my 21 years, that did not mean that I was the only one on the track. I used to see a couple of marathon runners at the high school track I worked out at in Memphis, usually on Tuesdays. Finally, one of them approached me and said "If we're going to be regulars here, we ought to know each other's names. I'm Darrell Croft." I later learned that he and his running mate were podiatrists, so when I developed heel spurs and plantar fasciitis in both feet in 2000, I knew who to call, and was well taken care of.

Another fellow that I met the same way was Bruce Babula M.D., an anesthesiologist and a distance runner. I never had to use his services, but we became good friends and still see each other from time to time when I'm in Memphis.

Even the coaches, both track and football, took note of my regularity and my purpose for being there. So when the school principal invoked a rule about outsiders not being welcome on the track, it was the assistant head football coach who showed me the easiest place in the fence to jump over when they weren't there to let me in.

And the list goes on. Nor do such meetings always take place at practice sessions. Since moving to Florida, the first 10 years I trained at the University of West Florida in Pensacola. After every Monday morning workout I would have lunch at Ci Ci's Pizza Parlor, on my way home. That's where I met Bill Spain, who had noticed that I came in regularly having apparently been working out in some fashion. He struck up a conversation which developed into weeks of friendly chit-chat, which later led to what no doubt kept me active in the game. I'll tell more about that in Chapters 12 and 15.

Family

On two occasions at the Tennessee state finals in Clarksville, my cousin Glenda and her husband, Jim Hartmann showed up unannounced, then again in Baton Rouge, Louisiana at the Nationals in 2001. And again in Norfolk, Virginia for the 2003 Nationals. And again in Biloxi, Mississippi in 2004 for the Gulf Coast Games. I tell you, folks, that kind of surprises can do wonders for your morale.

The next time I saw them at a meet was in Louisville, Kentucky for the 2007 Nationals. But this time they did not come just as spectators. Jim had decided in 2004 to get into the “swim” of things. Being from Pennsylvania he challenged his two brothers in a swim across the Monongahela River as a kickoff exercise for his getting into the Senior Games as a swimmer. And he’s still going strong.

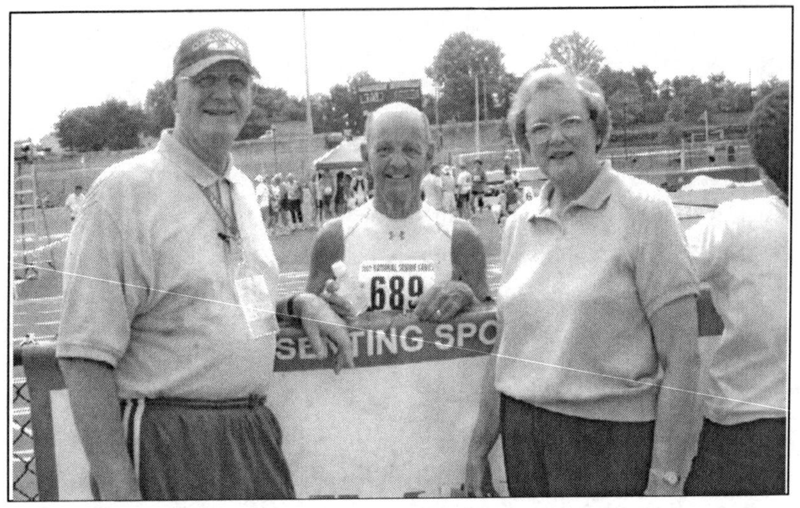

Senior Games National Championships, Louisville, KY 2007. John Hurd between cousin Glenda Hartmann and her husband, Jim. Jim had taken up swimming in The Games by this time.

12
And Then It Happened

In the 2000 Tennessee finals I won the 100m in World Class time, and made All American in both the 100m and 200m, but finished 2nd in the 200m and 400m. Yep, Jim Mathis had moved into my age group again. I never felt bad about finishing 2nd behind Jim, because he was truly in a class unto himself.

In 2001 the Nationals were held in Baton Rouge, Louisiana at the LSU track. At 69 I was the oldest man in the age group. Had it been run under current rules I would have been in the next higher age group, because I would be 70 before the year ended. But that is not what this chapter is about.

The afternoon temperature in Baton Rouge was 95 degrees on July 17, 2001. We had run the 100m two days earlier, in which they had confused the times between Don Beck and me. Nine of us had qualified the day before in the 200m prelims. We all did our warm-ups indoors where they had a short track. I started my stretches early to do a little extra and have time for my warm-up strides with some time left to relax before the 200m finals.

I had been on the floor on my back for most of the stretches. When I finished I jumped to a standing position and immediately began running in place with high knee lifts, at full speed. I was thinking this feels great; I'm going to have a really good run. Suddenly, with absolutely no warning, my gyroscope turned itself off. I found myself staggering with no control over anything but my consciousness. I tried to make it to the side of the room where there was a table to break my fall. I hit the deck in a sitting position, and before I could say what the heck happened there was an EMT on each of my arms. One was a female with her fingers on my right wrist checking my pulse, and the other male type was strapping a blood pressure cuff onto my left arm. I had fallen in front of the first aid booth. How about that!

I regained my footing and the EMTs helped me inside the booth where they ran an electrocardiogram (EKG) on me. One of them made a phone call and there was an M.D. cardiologist type on the scene in no time. I told him he would probably find a mitral valve prolapse (MVP) and a left bundle branch block (LBBB) on the chart, both of which he confirmed.

A quick flashback

In 1987 I had a series of anxiety attacks that I thought I had overcome 20 years earlier. I finally gave in and went for help. The doctor, James Boone M.D., prescribed three Xanax pills per day (tranquilizer) and a half pill of Tenormin, a beta block blood pressure medicine which, among other things, suppresses adrenaline. After six days of this I looked and felt like a walking zombie. Then I discovered that the pharmacist had put the labels on the wrong bottles. I was taking six times the amount of adrenaline suppressant that I should have been taking, and only 1/6th of the tranquilizer. When I called Dr. Boone to tell him about it, he told me to get right over to the pharmacy and show them the bottles. The lady pharmacist turned pale immediately when I showed them to her. I think I put her mind at ease by telling her I had no interest in a lawsuit; I just wanted to get well.

At my next physical checkup, a few months later, my EKG looked as though I had had a heart attack. The heart specialist described it as a change in the electrical conduction system. I later learned the name Left Bundle Branch Block (LBBB). Three years later Dr. Boone agreed with me that it was probably the pill mix-up that caused the condition.

Back to the Story Time Line

The doctor on the scene in Baton Rouge offered no opinion as to what brought about my tailspin, but at the advice of the EMTs, I scratched the 200m finals. I was not going to risk causing more of what I did not understand for a ribbon, then tell Sandy how dumb I was in doing so. I did go to see Doctor Boone when I got home and he opined that it was not a heart symptom. Twelve days after the incident I won the 100m and 200m events at the Tennessee finals, with John Wall right on my heels.

When something that sudden and that scary happens, one tends to look over one's shoulder lest it creep up on the scene again (at least this *One* continued to look for at least ten years). And on December 2nd of that year (2001) it did happen again, at the practice track. This time Dr. Boone took no chances and sent me to a cardiovascular clinic. They did the whole works: EKG, ECG (Echocardiogram, ultrasonic), 24 hour heart monitor, 30 day heart monitor, and even a drug induced stress test. I think they thought this 70 year old dude might not hold up under a treadmill test. On my next appointment they did put me on a treadmill, without notice. I was running in my socks and wound up with blisters on both feet.

When I passed all their tests and they still had no answers they wanted to implant a monitor into my left chest near the shoulder area. They thought the condition would get worse if I kept running and that I might be a candidate for a rapid heartbeat. Whoa, Nellie, as Keith Jackson used to say. I told my friend at the track, Dr. Bruce Babula, about all of this and he made out a list of questions to ask on my next appointment.

It was rather amusing, each time I checked in for an appointment. As soon as I would announce myself at the check-in counter, they would ask me for a list of my medicines. When I told them I did not take medicines, they would think I was being a smart aleck, and get agitated. For the record I have recorded 190 blood pressure tests for more than six years and the average is 121/65. The pulse average is 66, with a maximum of 78 and a minimum of 56. (Did I tell you that I still teach Microsoft Excel spreadsheet software at Pensacola State College (adjunct) and I am a compulsive score keeper?)

So I made another appointment just to talk, and that visit was just an oral Q&A session, just the cardiologist and me and a nurse who took notes. The bottom line was "You have never had a heart attack, you're not likely to die, and if it happens again, sit and rest for a few minutes." I think he suspected that he would never see me again, and he was right. "Goodbye, Doctor, and thank you."

All of that was comforting to know, but the uncomfortable thought that still lingered was that they did not know what happened, how to prevent it from happening again, or what to do about it if it did happen. So I continued with my training and competitions, but I must admit ~~that the~~ monkey was still hanging on my shoulder. I became rather tentative in my training, and in my warm-ups on game days.

A month after that session we had the Memphis games to qualify for the state. There were just four of us in our age group, Bob Alexander and two others that I never saw before or since. In the 100m, Bob was kind enough to lay back close to me so I would look somewhat respectable. We went through the motions, with me about half a second behind him, and a lady approached us afterward with “You guys were awesome.” Bob and I just smiled at each other, thinking that this sweet naïve lady doesn’t know point shaving when she sees it. Bob ran at his usual pace in the 200m and I was a good three seconds back. In the 400m we carried on a conversation around the entire oval. I almost had to push Bob over the finish line for him to beat me by .02 (2/100) of a second. I appreciated his concern, but an unearned gold medal was not what I signed on for.

Two months later we had the Tennessee finals. I felt OK, and won the 100m, 200m and 400m. In the 400m the man on my left was Fred Lovelace, M.D., so I thought it best to inform him of what could happen. “Fred,” I said, “If I get dizzy and fall, keep going. I’ll be alright.” Fred’s response was, “If you’re going to fall, do it in the other lane and don’t get in my way.” Who says anesthesiologists don’t have a sense of humor? (At least I think he was kidding.) I won and Fred finished second, ahead of Pastor Jim Tolbert and John Wall.

That same summer (2002) Sandy and I had picked out a lot in Navarre, Florida and construction had begun on our house. So In October, I drove down to check on the progress in Navarre, and took part in the local games in Pensacola, winning the 50m, 100m and 200m. That's the day we had to run the 50m a second time, because the man who finished second had jumped the gun. I had to win it twice because he took a flyer.

13
Florida, Here We Come

We moved to Florida in April, 2003. I had researched the Emerald Coast area from Pensacola to Panama City looking for tracks to train on. There were three: University of West Florida in Pensacola, 31 miles to the west; Destin Elementary School in Destin, 29 miles in the opposite direction; and Gulf Breeze High School, 15 miles to the west, and it was in ill repair. All the rest were paved with asphalt. We moved in on Saturday, I worked out at Gulf Breeze High School on Sunday, and Tuesday they were digging it up and repaving. This is going to be a lot of miles to drive four times a week. For ten years I drove the 31 miles each way to UWF, until they ripped theirs up in 2013 and repaved it. If the Destin Elementary School ever does that to their track, I guess I'll have to build my own track.

The Nationals were coming up in May of that year in Hampton Roads, Virginia, with track events in Norfolk. Sandy had never been able to travel with me to the Nationals before, because we would have to be gone for several days, and she had a job. So she took this opportunity to postpone job hunting and go to Norfolk with me. Also at the games were my cousins, Glenda and Jim Hartmann. I felt like I had groupies with me. It was really great.

I finished seventh in the 100m, and there was a man from Florida, Johnnie Morris, in fifth place .14 (14/100) of a second ahead of me. I would meet him again in the fall in the Florida state games. I finished fifth in the 200m, and don't remember why, but Morris was not in the finals.

The Florida games in ’03 were held in The Villages, Florida on December 6th. Believe it or not, the southern part of Florida can be cold in December. It was 41 degrees that morning and the wind must have been blowing at 41 knots. Besides my running shorts and singlet (shirt) I had my warm-ups on and a heavy hooded sweat-suit over all of that. And I kept them on until they called the 100m first call. Come on, folks, I moved to Florida to get warm.

There was Johnnie Morris again, the Florida favorite, and Thomas Phillips from Cincinnati, who had beaten both Morris and me in Norfolk. On this day they would settle for second and third place respectively, and neither of them started in the 200m. So I had the first of ten consecutive years of winning both the 100m and 200m dashes in Florida. In the results book, there was one man who won a single track event four years in a row, and that was the closest anyone else has come to my 10 year double since the Florida games began. My achievement is not officially recognized as a record, but to me it is.

The next year, 2004, John Wall and I met in Biloxi, Mississippi in April for the Mississippi Gulf Coast Senior Games. I won the 100m event in World Class and All American time, and John was a breath behind me. Warming up for the 200m I sprained an ankle. The first aid man on hand taped it really well for me and I decided to continue anyway, despite Sandy’s plea to use good common sense. But it had not begun to swell yet, so I promised her that if it did not work I would drop out immediately. It actually felt OK and I got another gold medal. The swelling and discoloration began later.

In September the Pensacola local games were cancelled, thanks to Hurricane Ivan. I called the authorities and asked about a qualification waiver for the state games, because the nearest alternative venue is Jacksonville, an eight hour drive away. "Sorry, you must qualify somewhere, and most of the other 17 venues have already completed their games." So I called Jacksonville and they accepted my late entry form and check.

Five days before the Jacksonville games I was finishing my workout, and ran a practice start with the starting blocks. I clipped off about 20 meters, turned to walk back, and had the dizzy problem again, falling against a fence. That was the last time I used the starting blocks.

On my way to Jacksonville I got a call from the authorities in the state office. They had approved my request for a qualification waiver. Ha. Thanks a lot, but I'd have to pay the motel anyway if I turned around now; besides I came to run and I'm almost there.

It turned out that my competition the next morning was Joe Hemler, the man who had won it all in San Antonio nine years earlier. Joe had been out of the game for some time, and was getting back into shape to run again. We were both starting from a standing position, but Joe knew how to do it. The gun went off and Joe flew off the line, while I was trying to get my balance. But Joe ran out of gas about half way down the track, and I overtook him. I have neither seen nor heard of him since then.

The 2004 Florida games were held in The Villages and in December again, as always. Six days before the games, I had another episode with the dizziness, falling into the bleachers on the last part of my warm-up drill. I did not finish the workout. With the games less than a week off I wanted to be sure that I was as ready as I could be.

I was still rather tentative in my pre-game warm-up at the Villages, but I did manage to win the 100m and 200m, though the times were not quite All American. Fortunately, I had achieved that level earlier in the year in Mississippi to keep my streak of eight years as an All American alive.

The next spring, of 2005, John Wall and I met again in the Mississippi Gulf Coast Games. I had been nursing an extremely sore left foot, just behind the 2nd and 3rd toes, counting from the big toe out. I had Googled, and had come across the term Morton's Neuroma, and looking up the word neuroma I came across the word tumor. Ain't no way I'm gonna have a doctor poking around that. So we ran the 100m dash, and John won it. I did not run the 200m, because it was really hurting after that.

So after I got back home I called around and found the name of a good orthopedic foot specialist and went to see Dr. Papacostas (probably Greek). I described my symptoms to him, and before I took my shoe and sock off he said "Nope, not Morton's. Wrong toe. Morton's is not a tumor, though it is similar in some ways. You have an inflamed metatarsal." So then I said to him, "I don't do pills, needles or knives." And he replied with those beautiful words, "No need. You're going to follow some stretches I've laid out." Cool. I can do that, and I began that afternoon following his directions. So help me, it was beginning to get better the next day. I kept the stretches up for several weeks, and have never had that problem again. He was my kind of doctor.

Two months later I went to Coral Springs, Florida, where the Masters were holding the Sunshine State championships, and won the 100m and 200m dashes. There I met two new friends, Norman and Violet Meeker, who happen to live 15 miles from me in Gulf Breeze. Norman is a middle distance runner and Vi is a tennis player in The Games and currently the state discus champion. Norman and I are sometimes in the same age group, but do not run in the same events. Both of them have accumulated several Florida state medals, and we've been good friends over the past 10 years.

My Only Florida Silver

In September of that year we had the Pensacola games, for qualifying for the state championships in December. That was 2005, right after hurricanes Dennis and Katrina showed up to finish whatever Ivan had left undone the year before. The result was that we did not have a properly surfaced track within 50 miles of Pensacola, so we had to run on the asphalt at Washington High School. They now have the only proper surface in the Pensacola area, but we are not privy to it for the games or for training. So I drive 28 miles in the other direction from Navarre to work out at the Destin Elementary School in Destin. But, let's get back to the games.

The 50m dash was the first event of the day, and starting from oldest to youngest, women then men, I was in the second heat. As I mentioned in chapter seven, I was so preoccupied with having to run on asphalt, and in flats, I paid no attention to the starter's commands or his rhythm with the gun in the first heat. We lined up, and I was expecting to hear the usual, "Runners to your marks," then "Get set," and then the sound of the gun. I had not noticed that the man didn't even have a gun. The only sounds I heard were "To your marks," then the weak toot of a toy horn. And while I looked around to see what the heck that was, everybody else took off. I don't know if you have ever run a 50m dash before, but 164 feet is not a long enough race to spot your opponents two or three steps before you start. When Bob Martin heard my footsteps near the end he strained so hard that he actually dove (unintentionally) over the finish line head first, ripping skin off his left arm and leg. The persons with the hand held stopwatches said Bob beat me by 1/100 of a second. Those tiny fractions matter, don't they? Bob earned the gold, I got the silver.

As banged up as he was, I couldn't believe Bob even felt like running the 100m, which came right after the 50m. But he did, and won the silver medal while I got the gold. In the 400m I must have felt like I had something to prove, because I actually sprinted the thing. I got another gold, but I was pooped and hoping for a little rest before the 200m. We ran all four of the events in less than an hour, on that hard pavement. To my good fortune, Bob did not enter the 200m, and I won the gold. But, as Tennessee Ernie Ford used to say, I felt like I'd been rode hard and put up wet. That's what running sprints on asphalt with heavy shoes and no spikes will do for you.

When we got to the state finals in December (2005), I had another minor disappointment. I was in my last year of the 70-74 age group and hadn't qualified for All American so far that year. I won the 100m again, edging Johnnie Morris out for the gold, but not in All American time. Then in the 200m, I was timed (electronically) at 32.01 seconds, and the qualifying time required was 32.00. When I picked up my gold medal and saw that time on the result sheet I moaned “Oh, no!” The lady at the table said, “Did we do something wrong?” “No ma’am,” I said, “I did.”

So my streak of All American status every year ended by 1/100th of a second after eight years, but my streak of consecutive wins in both the 100m and 200m in the State Finals was just beginning at three years.

The following May of 2006, I entered the State Finals in Clinton, Mississippi and we had a Tennessee reunion. Bob Alexander was there from Memphis and John Wall from Cookeville. Bob won the 50m in 8.44 seconds, John got the silver in 8.51, and I got a bronze with 8.54. There was no All American standard for the 50m, because it was not part of the National games, and many states did not have it either. In the 100m, I took the gold with 14.75 seconds, which was All American and World Class time. Bob got the silver with 15.13 seconds, and John got the bronze with 16.52 seconds. In the 200m Bob outlasted me for the gold at 31.02 to 31.18, John came in 3rd at 33.82, and all three of us were in All American times.

I must mention that even though John, Bob and I took the gold, silver and bronze medals, the Mississippi contestants in 4th place and below also received medals in each race as though we were not there.

Enter Only the Events You Trained For

In September we held the Pensacola games, where we qualify for the State Finals. I won the 50m, 100m, 200m and 400m and proceeded toward the parking lot with my gear, when I got a bad case of curiosity. As I passed by the long jump area, they were preparing to hold the standing long jumps. I didn't know there was such an event, so I set my bag down and put my name on the roster. They're pretty good about that in Florida at the local and state events.

Well, I jumped as far as I could, 7 feet 0 inches, which was good enough to win. But I paid for it for over a year. I pulled a groin muscle, the adductor, and could barely walk the next two days. Take my advice and stick to the script.

At the State Finals in December I won both the 100m and 200m dashes in All American time. The 200m record was 33.16 seconds for the 75-79 age group, and I ran it in 32.66 seconds. I felt that setting a new record pretty much made up for not making All American the previous year.

14
Never Was a Hoss

...that couldn't be rode. Never was a cowboy that couldn't be throwed.

I still hadn't completely recovered from the pulled groin muscle, and I was still paying for it months later after weeks of ultra-sound and massage therapy.

Meanwhile, one month before the national games in Louisville, Kentucky in 2007, I had two of the dizzy spells back to back after my warm-up stretches. I thought maybe it was time to give the conventional medical system another opportunity to find out what was causing it. After getting my records from the heart specialists in Memphis, I was sent to a neurologist to continue the mystery of why it happens. He ruled out vertigo, but did call for more tests, including a brain scan which indicated nothing was wrong there.

So when it came time to prepare for the trip to the National games I hadn't trained that well and really didn't want to go. But my inner voice, aka my conscience, my cheerleader, my strongest supporter, my bride Sandy, took her position as always. She said "You've been going every two years, hoping to get a medal, and coming home with fifth and seventh place ribbons. You didn't go to Pittsburgh in '05 because of a sore foot. This may be the year you will actually get a medal." And I said "Yeah, but if this adductor muscle acts up, I might not even qualify for the finals." And she said "I don't care if you don't even suit up. Go and be with your friends, enjoy yourself, and make that decision after you get there." And so I went to Louisville. Wouldn't every man love to have that kind of support at home?

As I walked out to the track for the first day's event, the 100 meter dash preliminary, George Spero, another of my Tennessee friends, approached me before I set my gear down. He was nursing a sore hamstring and told me they wanted me to fill in for him in the 4x100 meter relay. We had always talked about getting a Tennessee group together if they ever held relay competitions. I was excited about the request, but I had to tell him they might want to wait until after the 100 meter dash before they got excited too. So we ran the 100 meter preliminaries, and for the first (and only) time since my first national trip in 1995, I did not make the finals. The top nine finishers qualified, and I had the 11th best time.

I have to admit that the next morning I was a bit depressed. I had pretty much slipped into a comfort zone of placing between fifth and seventh place in the 100m and 200m dashes at the national events, and today I was a spectator. But my two good Tennessee buddies, John Wall and Bob Alexander had finished fifth and seventh respectively in the 100m and we asked another Tennessee friend, Charlie Baker, to complete the foursome with us. Charlie was five years older than I was, and had won the silver in his age group. I felt really good about the foursome, and with a day of rest my mood quickly recovered.

The next morning we had the 200 meter prelims, and I had the sixth best time to qualify for the finals the next day. Two hours later we lined up for the 4x100 meter relay. Bob would lead off, because he was fast out of the blocks. He would hand it to me coming out of the first turn, I would then take it to Charlie, and he would round the next curve and hand it to John for the anchor leg. We were in lane 1.

Bob Alexander's other persona is body builder. He looks like something in a text book on body building or sprinting. But standing in that narrow 44 inch wide lane he looked like a runaway train coming straight for me. I felt like jumping out of the way. But I took my position and he handed me the baton and I delivered it to Charlie Baker, who gave it to John Wall. By the time John crossed the finish line with it he was a full 25 meters (4.25 seconds) ahead of the nearest man to him. All four of us had won a gold medal. It was not an individual win, but it was gold and it was my first medal at the national level. The next day I won the fifth place ribbon in the 200 meter finals and I was one happy boy. (At 75 I still thought of myself as a boy. In fact I still do at 83.) Sandy was right. I guess that's why they say "Some you win, some you lose, and some are rained out. But you suit up for every game." To that I add "We came to run, so let's run."

The winners in the 100m finals were Harry Brown from IL, Don Cheek (CA), Joe Summerlin (TX), Jim Stookey (MD), John Wall (TN), Frank Welch (AZ), Bob Alexander (TN), Lee Alexander (NE) and Al Raynor (FL). In the 200m it was again Harry Brown, Don Cheek, Joe Summerlin in the first three spots, followed by Bob Alexander, John Hurd, John Wall, Frank Welch and Bill Wareham (TX). Remember those first three names in each race. We will meet again.

In May of 2008 I entered the Alabama State Finals in Montgomery and won the 100m and 200m dashes in All

American times. Later that year the Pensacola track and field games were cancelled in September because of budget constraints. At about the time they would have happened I had another dizziness attack while chasing a baby lizard that had sneaked into the house.

This time I was granted a waiver for local qualifying, and I did win the 100m and 200m events at the Florida State Finals, again in All American times. I was still in the process of learning how to start from a standing position, but I ran well and felt great.

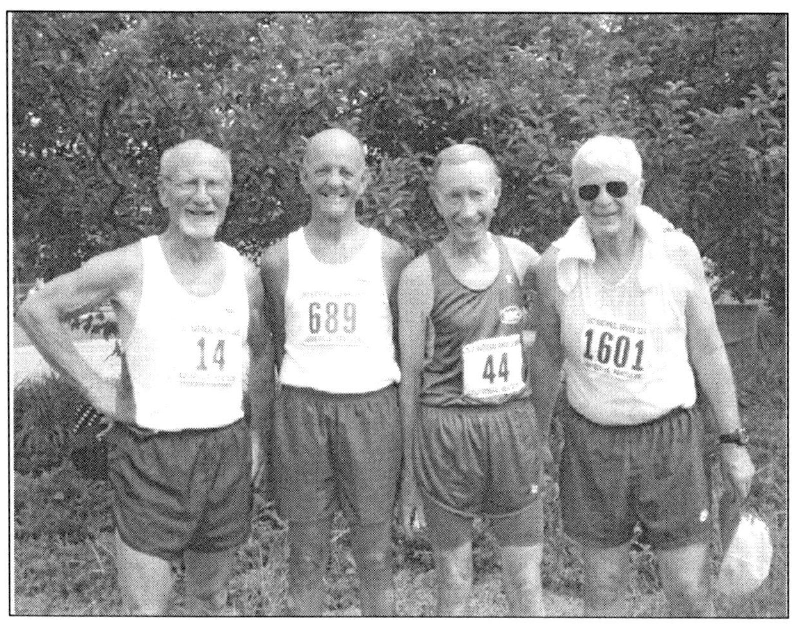

My first medal at the national level – age 75-79, 4 x 100 meter relay, Gold, time 63.93 seconds, Senior Games National Championships, Louisville, Kentucky June 28, 2007. Left to right: Bob Alexander, Memphis, TN, John Hurd, formerly Memphis, TN now Navarre, FL, Charlie Baker, Hixson, TN, John Wall, Cookeville, TN.

15
Time to Get Help

Flashback

Shortly after moving to Florida, around 2005 or 2006, Sandy and I were visiting our friends Edgar and Jean Buffaloe who had moved from Memphis to Panama City Beach in 2002. When I told them about the experiences with dizziness, Edgar told me it was in my neck. Being a natural skeptic, I muttered something like "yeah, right." Then he said, "Johnny, if you're having dizzy problems, I guarantee you it's in your neck." He then felt the back of my neck and told me my atlas was out of alignment. I didn't know an atlas from a barbell, and had no idea he had gone to chiropractic school years before. And I learned that the atlas is the first vertebra at the base of the skull.

On April 30, 2007 I was having lunch at my favorite Monday restaurant, Ci Ci's Pizza, after working out, when the man across the aisle struck up a conversation. His name was Bill Spain and he had seen me there many times and was aware that I had probably been working out. He was a runner and very knowledgeable about food supplements. We had a few weekly conversations, and one day he asked me to e-mail him some information I had on goji berry juice. When he gave me his card with his e-mail address I learned that he was Dr. Bill Spain, MS, DC, CCSP, a chiropractor.

I asked Dr. Spain if there was any validity to what Edgar had told me about my atlas causing the dizzy spells, and he assured me there was. There is a major artery passing though each side of the atlas that sends blood to the base of the brain. When the vertebra gets off center, it naturally squeezes the arteries and suppresses blood flow, and one can become dizzy. Made sense to me.

Back to 2009

On April 2, 2009 I arrived at the UWF track for my workout. I set my bag down and started to the restroom. It had been raining, and I took a small jump over a puddle, got dizzy, and did a nosedive into the grass. When I regained my balance, I picked up my bag and went back to the car. I called Sandy to tell her I was coming home, and she gave me very explicit instructions. I had a strong feeling that this was not a suggestion. She told me to call Dr. Spain and make an appointment - *now*. So I did, and on April 7th he x-rayed me, adjusted me, and had his massage therapist work my neck and shoulders. He asked me to give him 90 days, and so I did. I was still seeing him regularly, though not as often, until he retired in the summer of 2014. Before he left he introduced me to Dr. Amanda Gottschalk, whom I see now in Ft. Walton Beach. So he left me in good hands, literally.

Dr. Spain likes to call me his poster boy. He tells me that most men my age are sitting around the TV watching reruns of *Gilligan's Island*. And really, folks, that and the friends and fun and staying off the couch and out of drugstores and doctors' offices are what it's all about.

Since that first appointment, almost six years ago, I have not had one recurrence of the dizziness that goes by the name "syncope." Thank you, Edgar Buffaloe, for directing me to Dr.

Bill Spain. And thank you, Dr. Spain, for helping me stay in The Game.

And The Beat Goes On

In the Pensacola games in September of 2009, I won the 50m in World Class time, and both the 100m and 200m in All American time. Sandy thought it would be good for me to spread out and get more game experience, so two weeks later I headed for Baton Rouge, Louisiana for a weekend of their state championships. When I drove onto the campus at LSU, I was reminded of the unpleasant experience I had there in 2001, with the dizziness. I felt like I was getting back on the horse that threw me. But all went well, and I took the 50m, the 100m, and I won the 200m in All American time. Fortunately, my Louisiana friend Charley Richard (pronounced Re shard') is younger and had not entered my age group yet.

The Florida State Championships were held in Ft. Myers in December again, and I was fortunate enough to win my two dashes, the 100m and 200m. The 50m event would not be introduced at the state level in Florida for three more years.

Recognition Time

In April of 2010 I had a special treat. The Pensacola Sports Association recognized five of us senior athletes from the Pensacola area with a Special Achievement Award at their annual awards banquet. Norman Meeker, Roger Dobson, Dan Keely, Dennis Seaman and I had all won state championships the previous December. Dennis won his in field events, and the rest of us are runners or sprinters.

Norman has authored a book about his adventures with tanks in the Korean War, titled *Shouting On the Way,* available on Amazon.com. (Really, I think his main reason for writing the book was to tell how he met, in Japan, his lovely wife Violet, nee Misako Yokoyama.) He included a picture of the four of us runners, which he likes to call "four pretty fast seniors." Roger is the father of Matthew Dobson, who helps coordinate our local events and serves as starter for the running events. Dan Keely is the retired cross country coach of The University of West Florida.

The awards banquet was really a first class affair, and I don't think I had ever heard the words All American used so many times in one evening.

In May of 2010 I went back to Clinton, Mississippi for their annual state championships. I won the 100m dash in All American time, the 50m in World Class time, and also won the 200m event.

For the Pensacola games in September, the UWF track was not available, so we had the meet at Catholic High School. Since hurricanes Ivan, Dennis and Katrina had done their number on their rubberized track surface, they had ripped the cover off and repaved it with asphalt. Shortly after we moved to Florida in 2003, Andrews Institute, a large orthopedic clinic, opened facilities in Gulf Breeze. I believe their market research must have projected a lot of business from all the asphalt tracks on The Emerald Coast.

In the Florida state championships in December, I won both the 100m and 200m dashes for the eighth year in a row. I don't think many records were set that day in the sprints, because of the headwinds. In the 200m, it showed -7.4 on the official wind gauge, which means the wind was in our face at the speed of 7.4 meters per second, or about 16.6 miles per hour. When you're running 14 to 16 mph, that's a total force of over 30 mph.

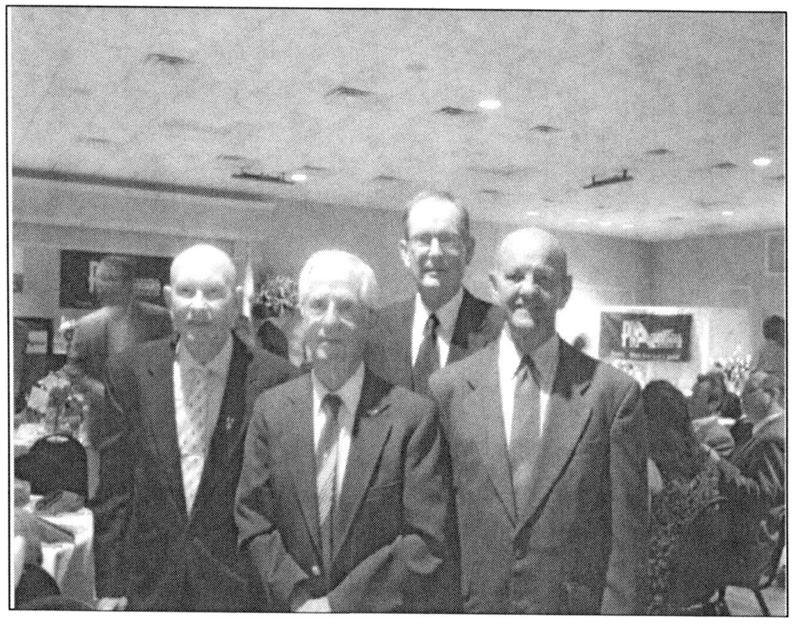

L to R Norman Meeker, Dan Keely, Roger Dobson, John Hurd, recipients of Special Achievement awards by the Pensacola Sports Association for Florida state championships in track events in 2009. Norman likes to call this picture "Four Pretty Fast Seniors."

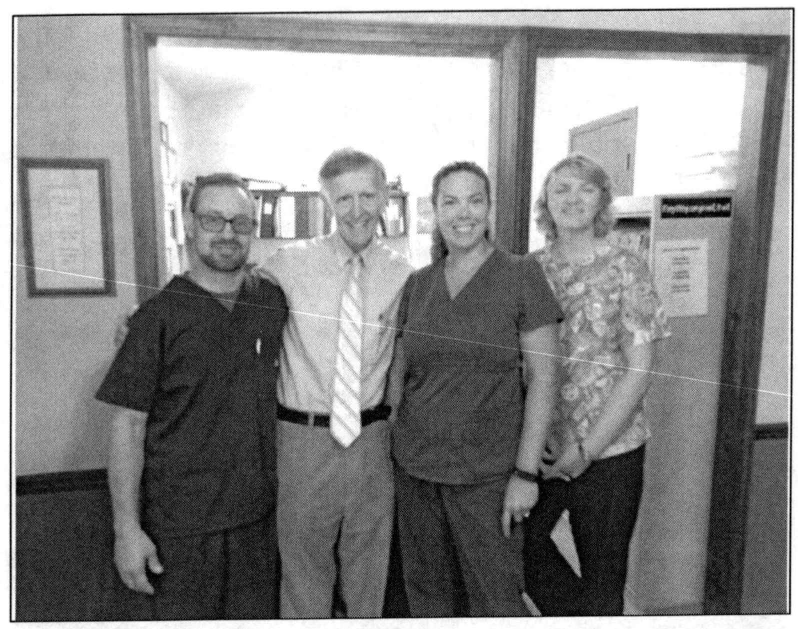

The man who corrected the dizzy spells and kept me in The Games, Dr. Bill Spain, MS, DC and his staff. Left to Right: Will Funches, Licensed Massage Therapist, Dr. Spain, Dr. Amanda Gottschalk, DC and Cindy Mulvey, Receptionist.

16
2011 – Nationals in Humble, Texas

I had skipped the national games in San Francisco in 2009. I had pretty much given up flying in 1980 (unless Sandy was traveling with me), and that would have been a more than 5,000 mile round trip drive with several nights in motels. Now the 2011 games were coming up, in the Houston, Texas area.

Before I get into this part of the story, I feel I should give you some idea of my mindset at the time. Sandy and I had been (and still are) attending a semi-annual gathering of the *Core Living* group. It's about 100 friends who meet in Howell, Michigan (yes, we fly there) where Jerry McLean, multi-millionaire businessman who formerly played hockey with the Detroit Wings, donates his time and his knowledge to share with us some principles of living that are invaluable to us. One thing that I was made aware of was that my dream of someday winning an individual medal in the national games had been just that – a dream. Before this trip, I converted that dream to a goal with a date on it.

There were three men who were perennial favorites to take the top three medals. This would be the same three I wrote about in Chapter 14, saying that we would meet again later. It's now later. One of those three was Joe Summerlin from the Houston area. Joe and I had been competing with each other for years, and he had been beating me like a rented mule all those years. We had become close friends, even though we only saw each other every two years at most. My goal was to share the winner's podium (top three) along-side Joe, no matter what color the medal was. To do that I'd have to beat either Don Cheek from California or Harry Brown from Illinois, neither of whom I had ever beaten before. And nobody was beating Harry.

There were several people entered in my age group, so that we had to run the 100 meter event three times in two days. In the preliminaries, I had this foolish idea that I could qualify without having to exert too much in this first heat, until I glanced to my left and saw Sonny Oliphant from Mississippi moving up. Game on! I managed to win that one, and qualified for the semi-finals to be run later in the day.

Joe Summerlin and I were in adjacent lanes for the semi-finals that afternoon, and we all had to go for broke to be sure to qualify for the finals the next day. I had been starting from a stand-up position since the experience with dizziness in Baton Rouge in 2001, 10 years before. So Joe got out ahead of me, as usual, but I caught him at the finish line. For the only time I have ever seen it happen, they had to go to three decimal places to determine the winner of our heat. Joe won it by one thousandth of a second, 16.394 to 16.395. As we crossed the finish line Joe turned to his left and said "What are you doing?" He had never seen me up close before in a race. We were both laughing, and we both qualified for the finals. The only casualty of the race was that the sole of one of my track shoes had broken all the way across on the bottom.

We were supposed to run the 100 meter finals the next morning, Tuesday, at 10:00 AM. It rained the entire day, which was bad enough, but there was also lightning and thunder throughout. Every time it would thunder, which of course meant lightning, we had to go hide under the stands until 30 minutes had passed without another occurrence. We wound up doing our warm-ups four different times, and didn't get to run until after 1:00 PM. We had no lunch, and I'm a guy who doesn't do anything without getting fed on time. It was still raining hard while we watched the 80-84 year old ladies ahead of us wait patiently with rain in their faces, and run their heat. Remember that comment I made about some games being rained out? That does not apply in track events.

We finally got off, and as usual I was behind all three of them. But I was determined to get one of those medals, so I had to pass either Joe or Don. I finally caught up with them at about the 75 or 80 meter mark, and POW! My right hamstring felt like a spear had hit it. I hollered out loud.

One of the things I had learned in Jerry McLean's *Core Living* gatherings was that when facing a major decision, the first quarter of a second is very crucial. I later calculated that in a quarter of a second I would travel about five feet, which is a huge gap in a 100 meter race. So I didn't have time to think about whether I was going to take a dive, or pull up to save myself, or to continue and possibly cause more damage to the muscle. My only thought was "I'm in second place, and I'm going to get a medal." I poured more coals on the fire, and never broke stride.

Harry shattered the record, and by the time the rest of us crossed the finish line it seemed as if he had been finished for quite a while. Having heard me holler, he had already turned around and was on his way back to help me. I was hurting, but as Broadway Joe Willie Namath once said, "When you're winning, nothing hurts."

Harry didn't just tell me where the first-aid room was, he was helping me limp to the other end of the track. But I had to wait and ask Joe how he did. "Joe, did you get second?" I asked. With what seemed like excitement in his voice and on his facial expression he answered "No, you did." Joe was third. That, dear readers, is what the games are all about. You feel like you'd run through hot coals to beat as many of the others as you can, but when it's over you still remember that you're good friends first.

So Harry and I made it to the first-aid room and got me iced up. Then I had to call Sandy and give her the good and bad news. It went something like this: "Hi Honey. I earned my first individual national medal and it will be silver, but I may be home early." Then I related the whole day's experiences to her: the rain, the lightning, the thunder, the multiple warm-ups, the three hour delay with nothing to eat, the doubt about the 200 prelims tomorrow morning, and my sore leg.

She was naturally excited about the medal and disappointed about the leg, but she was nowhere near ready to hear about my giving up. She "encouraged" me to seek any help I could find – a physical trainer or massage therapist or anybody that could help get me back in the game by tomorrow. So I agreed to continue the icing at the motel, and see how the warm-up goes in the morning. By starting time at 9:00 AM I would either be warmed up and waiting by the starting line or watching from the spectators' bleachers.

I got to the track a little early Wednesday morning, eager to see how my leg was going to behave. Another thing that Jerry has taught us to do in making decisions, is to ask ourselves

"What do I know for sure?" I made it through the warm-ups OK, except for the leg swings and the quick start, so I knew I would skip both of those. Despite the soreness, it didn't seem to have an adverse effect on my running. So I also knew I was going to run. I spoke to another Texas friend, Wayne Bennet, and confided that I was going to have to forego trying to be the first one off the line at the gun. Wayne is a few years younger than I am, so he is not in my age bracket, and has been competing much longer than I have, with a lot of wins and a Texas Hall of Fame on his resume. His advice was to wait and accelerate in the curve. Remember, the 200 meter dash is one half the distance around the oval track, covering most of the curve in the first 90 meters or so.

So, what did I know for sure? I knew four things for sure:

1. I knew that the pain was present when I did the leg swings, so I did not do them in my warm-up.
2. I knew the pain was also present when I did a fast start, so I had to be patient at the start and give it all I had on the curve and the ensuing straightaway.
3. I knew the leg was doing well at a semi-competitive pace, and with luck it would hold at top speed.
4. With that, I knew that I still had a good shot at a medal.

There were six heats in the preliminaries, with as many as eight runners in each heat. The top eight best times would determine the qualifiers for the finals, regardless of your position in your heat. By good fortune, I was in the last heat, so I could see what I had to do to be one of the eight. I counted and memorized the best eight times before my heat, so I knew the time I had to beat to qualify. I ran well enough to get the fifth best time, while Harry, Joe and Don finished in that order for the top three times. My Tennessee friend, John Wall, had the ninth best time, but since they had moved the venue from The University of Houston, we were on a track that only had eight lanes, so John didn't get to continue.

Meanwhile, we had another 4x100 meter relay event coming this same afternoon. Bob Alexander had retired from the games several months earlier for health reasons, so we recruited Dick Chapin from Montana. Dick had actually run relays before, and was a big help in showing us a good technique for exchanging batons. Dick led off, John Wall ran the second leg, Charlie Baker ran the third, and I ran the anchor leg. We finished ahead of the second place team by 12.82 seconds (about 71 meters or 78 yards), and I had my second national gold medal, both having come through the relays.

Suddenly it was Thursday, and time for the 200 meter finals. Our timing positions in the prelims determined the lanes we would be in for the finals on Thursday. Our lane assignments worked out to be exactly the way I would have asked for them. Joe Summerlin was in lane five and almost out of sight because of the stagger around the curve. Harry Brown was in lane four, Don Cheek was in lane three, and I was in lane two. Most sprinters prefer lanes other than one or two, because of the torque on the tight turns. With my short legs, that never was much of a concern to me. Besides, from here I could keep my eye on the big three and, coming out of the curve I would know where I stood. Of course, there was someone in each of the eight lanes, but these were the ones of major concern to me.

I may have mentioned before that I count things, even the steps I take when I run. On this day my mind was focused on something else entirely. From the crack of the gun, my one thought that I kept repeating to myself, was "I'm gonna beat Don Cheek, I'm gonna beat Don Cheek." I had no awareness of the soreness in my right leg, as it was performing well. As we got past the 150 meter mark I could see that I had a chance to catch up. My mantra changed to "I'm passing Don Cheek, I'm passing Don Cheek." And I did! I crossed the finish line well behind Harry, who had destroyed another record, but one tenth of a second ahead of Don, and a bit more ahead of Joe, who had apparently strained a hip muscle.

I think Joe and Don were so intent on beating Harry that they exhausted themselves, while I was forced to run a more balanced pace. Or as Commander Spock might have said, "Random factors seem to have operated in my favor." Anyway, I felt lucky. Later, after we had received our medals, Wayne Bennett, who had won many national medals, commented that he thought that this year's medals were gaudy. These two silvers were my first individual medals I had earned at the national level, and I thought they were beautiful. "Wayne," I said, "I love gaud."

In the Pensacola local games in September I won the 50m and both the 100m and 200m in All American times. Then in December I repeated the 100m and 200m wins at the state finals for the ninth consecutive year, and qualified for All American honors in both of them.

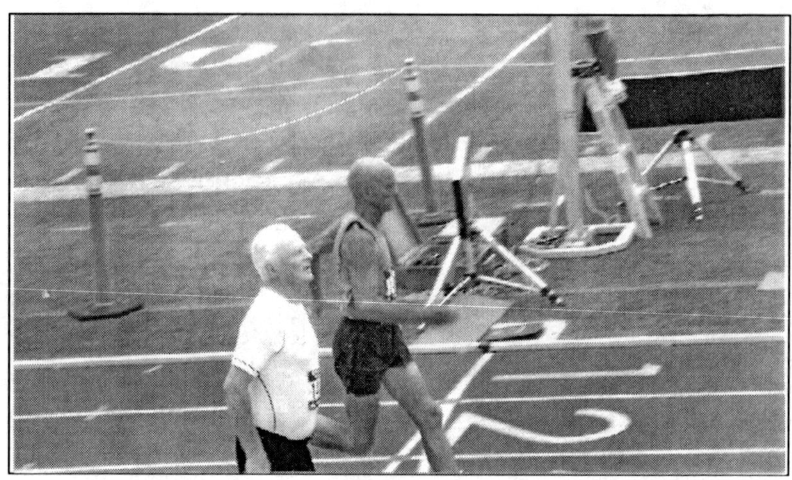

This is what one thousandth of a second looks like. Left to right: Joe Summerlin, Spring, TX, John Hurd, Navarre, FL, 100 meter semi-final of the Senior Games National Championships in Humble, TX June 21, 2011. Joe won the heat; his time was 16.394 seconds, mine was 16.395. Photo courtesy of Dora Yates.

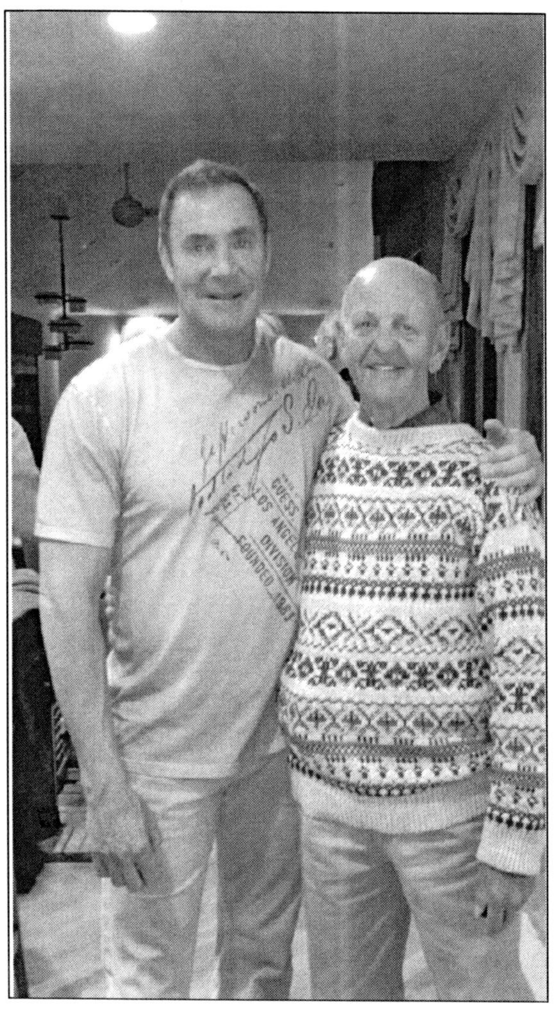

Jerry McLean of Core Living, and me at the "Gathering."

17
2012 – I Met the Man

In April of 2012 I went back to Clinton, Mississippi for their state games. I wanted to qualify for the 2013 nationals and it's good to keep active for the experience and the conditioning. I enjoy the games there, because the people are very friendly and they have a get-together dinner with live music the night before the track and field events.

Usually I'm very relaxed at these out of state meets, because other than qualifying for the next year's nationals, it's just good training. However, at the social gathering the evening before the games I met a fellow sprinter in my age group I had not known before named Perry Huff. It turned out that Perry had gone to the San Francisco national games that I skipped in 2009, and had come home with a gold medal and a silver one. Uh-oh! I've got to be on my toes tomorrow.

The next morning we had a cold, vicious headwind. Some of the sprinters were running in warm-ups or sweat-suits. But we had a good meet and I managed to win the 50m in 9.05 seconds, the 100m in 16.98, and the 200m in 35.64. Both the 100m and 200m were All American times.

When the 55-59 age group of women lined up for the 100m race, I noticed that one of them was using a modified three-point starting position without blocks. When the gun sounded she took off like a rocket, and finished well ahead of the pack. I watched her again in the 200m, and she repeated the performance. I was impressed. She had apparently had some good coaching.

I later spotted the lady sitting in the grass resting, and struck up a conversation. We exchanged compliments for a while, which made me feel really good. She said that her husband was a trainer, and mentioned the phrase “Ready Set Go!” that they used in their running. That was the title of a book I had studied for years, so I piped up with “Yeah, I know that book well; it was written by Phil Campbell from Jackson, TN. It’s all about high intensity workouts which increase the body’s human growth hormone by several hundred percent.” I knew that he had trained thousands of athletes at his training camp, from children to pro football players from the NFL. I was really sounding knowledgeable, or so I thought.

As we finished our conversation I introduced myself and asked her name. She said, “I’m Cathy Campbell.” And I unconsciously said, “You said your husband is here too. What’s his name?” She said “Phil. He’s Phil Campbell.” Duh!!! The author of the book I was trying to sound so up on. Boy, did I feel stupid! But my excitement totally overcame that feeling immediately. “I’ve got to meet him,” I blurted. She offered to be sure that I would meet him before I left.

After I finished all my events and got all my stuff together, I strolled around looking for Phil Campbell and spotted a man I thought I recognized from his picture in his book. He was talking with some other men. Ten yards away Cathy was talking to a couple of women. After a polite brief wait I called over impolitely to Cathy and asked “Is that Phil over there?” She said “Yes it is. Phil, that’s the man I was telling you about.” Phil looked around and answered “Hey, he’s the man I was telling *you* about.” And I was thinking “We’re going to get along really well.”

I walked up and introduced myself, and he began to tell me what good running form I had and I naturally ate it up. After a few more exchanges of compliments we posed for a picture of the three of us with my phone. Phil then said that if I didn't mind giving him my mailing address he'd like to send me his newest training DVD, *Run Your Fastest 40 Ever*. I told him that would be a lot of trouble to go to just for a free DVD. NOT!!! I dug a pen and pad out of my gear bag so quickly he didn't see where it came from.

About three days after I got home, a package came for me. It contained not just the DVD, but also the latest update of his book *Ready Set Go!*. Don't you love it when somebody says he'd like to send you so-and-so, and as soon as he gets home he actually sends that, and more? And without an invoice!

The video was full of excellent training tips, stretches, and of course the starting technique that I had seen Cathy use. But even though Dr. Spain's treatments of the misaligned atlas that caused the dizzy spell in Baton Rouge 11 years before had given me three full years without another incident, I was still reluctant to risk coming up from ground level suddenly at the pistol firing.

So in September at the Pensacola games I was still starting from a standing position, and won the 100m and 200m in All American times, and the 50m in World Class time. And the next chapter was a whirlwind of excitement for me.

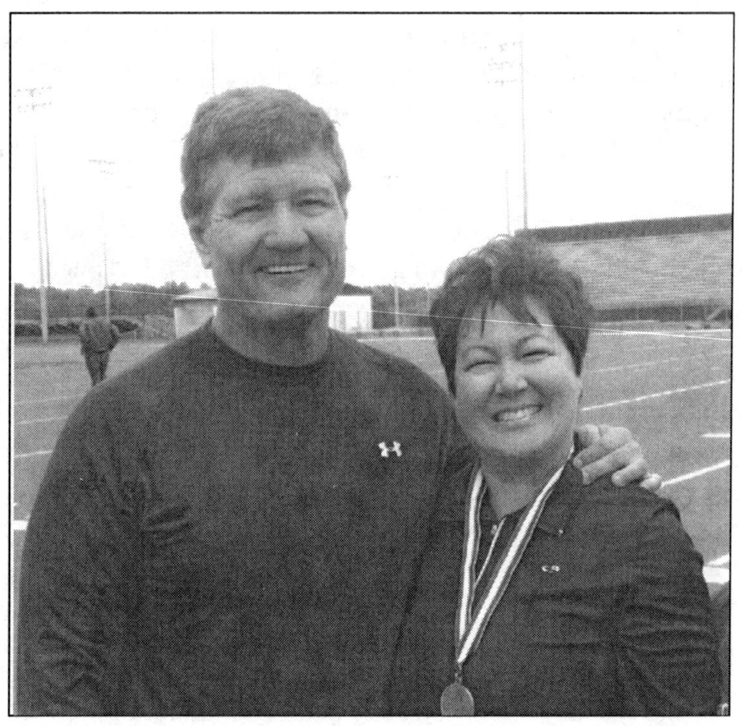

Phil & Cathy Campbell. Phil is the author of the book *Ready, Set, Go! - Synergy Fitness for Time-Crunched Adults..*

18
Into The Hall - My Fifteen Minutes

I had attended a Memphis Amateur Sports Hall of Fame annual induction celebration in 2002 with my friend Edgar Buffaloe (the non-practicing chiropractor who diagnosed my neck condition), when he accepted the posthumous award for Rye Ridblat, his boxing coach of many years.

Edgar was the classiest boxer with the fastest hands I had ever seen. He had a total of 76 fights in the ring, and never lost a decision, or even got knocked down. He did lose three of them, not by decision, but because he would break hand bones or re-injure the last such incident, but he never got out-boxed.

When Edgar's Naval squadron of F4U Corsairs got called to active duty in July of 1950, they sent them to southern California for combat training. In the first two months he was there Edgar put on 14 pounds. As a result, he moved up two weight divisions from featherweight to welterweight, and won the Pacific Fleet boxing championship.

The following year Edgar was training for the next tournament. One day, after he had just finished his workout, a stranger asked him if he would spar a couple of rounds with him. Edgar was already tired from his own workout, but reluctantly agreed.

After the first round, Edgar's buddy, Gene Harrison, told him he'd better step it up a bit, because the guy was getting to him. Edgar said "I have news for you, Gene. I did step it up. This guy is good." After the second and last round, Edgar said to the man, "If you're going to be in this upcoming tournament, I'd like to know that now!" "Oh, no" the fellow answered, "I'm a professional fighter. My name is Willie Pep." Holy Moly! Willie Pep was the featherweight champion of the world! He had been Edgar's idol for years.

Edgar clipped an article from a newspaper a few days later where Pep was asked who he thought was the next contestant worthy of challenging him for his title. His answer was "The best I've seen lately was an amateur sailor here in California named Ed Buffaloe."

So, I talked to my good friends Alex McCollum (ex-husband of my first wife, Gwen) and Larry Hilbun about getting Edgar nominated in the boxing category. To me, it seemed to be a given that if the Memphis Hall of Fame had a boxing category at all, Edgar should be in it.

Alex McCollum had been the Mid-South heavyweight Golden Gloves champion himself, but was a member of the Hall of Fame in the basketball category. Larry Hilbun was entered in the fast pitch softball category as a pitcher and both of them have also served terms as president of the Hall of Fame association. At that time they didn't have a category yet for track and field.

It's ten years later, now 2012, and I got a call from Larry. A track and field category had just been added a year or two earlier, and Alex had submitted my name this year in nomination for membership. Larry was going to prepare and present my dossier to the nominating committee and he wanted all pertinent data, including news stories and anything that would give the members what they would need to make their decisions. Since I have recorded every event and the results of every meet I've been in, on a spreadsheet, it took me a very short time to put that together for him.

After what seemed like years, Larry called and then Alex called to tell me I had been selected to be inducted on December 3rd as a member of the Memphis Amateur Hall of Fame for 2012. I got excited!

I'll let Sandy, my bride, tell you what happened next. Here's Sandy.

First, we had to put together a list of names and addresses for the invitations. Nothing quite like this had ever happened to John before, and we wanted everybody who might be interested, to know about it, whether they could come or not. Larry was a big help with the addresses of fraternity brothers that he hadn't seen in years.

Then I, Sandy, decided there had to be a party the next day for those who came to the award banquet, and for those who for some reason could not make it. So I prevailed upon John's brother Walker to "volunteer" his home for an open house the evening after the main event. He was a pushover for the idea, as usual. You see, Walker's friend Sherry McClure, has just helped him completely re-decorate his house and it has become "the place" for every family party, shower, or anything else. Walker says he's fine as long as you clean up! What a transformation it has been and Sherry is responsible for the decoration part. Walker just provided the money and said OK a lot! It is magnificent!

We had to reach everyone quickly so they could save the dates on their calendars, so we compiled a list of everyone's e-mail addresses we could find and then mailed a copy of the e-mail to people for whom we only had mailing addresses. I then contacted all of the nieces, Janis Hurd Twilley, Susan Lewis, Sherry Campbell, nephew Jimmy Lowery and sister Jo Lowery, and any daughters-in-law in the family (it's a big family) and asked them to assist with food or beverages. In order to keep the house a comfortable temperature, we decided to restrict the foods to things that required no oven.

Next, I enlisted my two friends here in Florida, where we live now, Iris Lawrence and Cindy Hibbard, to help from this end. We three have planned and executed more things than you can imagine and all three are creatively talented and each has her own niche. It always turns out great!

Iris decided she would provide the congratulatory cake and decorate the cake table with special candles and candlesticks and Cindy would assist with staging all of the picture and plaque awards on the window seat in the dining room where Walker lives. Sandy would coordinate everything and find a way to display all of the 99 gold medals that had been won. Sherry Mac came through with a wrought iron Christmas tree wrapped with lights up the center and she created a beautiful red bow on top from red mesh fabric. There were red, white and blue Christmas balls on the tree and then on the day of the party, son, John Jr. helped me tie all of the medals with red, white and blue ribbons on the tree. We even hung the three most important ones from the chandelier over the food table.

Son, John Jr. had driven down to Memphis from Baltimore, MD to be there for both evenings. He is so creative himself! He has completely re-done his beautiful Antique Row House in Baltimore. We saw pictures and it is just incredible what he can do and has done!

We enlisted Rhonda Hurd, Walker's daughter-in-law, to provide the dishes for the table, as with three of us in the car and all of the medals and awards, suitcases and clothes, there would be no more room for dishes! She was happy to oblige! Rhonda does some catering herself, so she had everything we needed.

Now that we had things going in the right direction, I made a list of foods that we could get from Sam's Club to add the finishing touches to the food table. Iris and I shopped our local Sam's to get the prices so when we arrived in Memphis, we could get things we needed quickly.

Finally the day arrived to head to Memphis. We had told Cindy and Iris they could only have one small suitcase, so they brought their suitcases over so we could see if we could fit everything into our Toyota Camry. It was a tight squeeze, but we decided we could put our outfits for the two occasions on top of everything else in hanging bags. Packing the car was hilarious! By the time we got everything in, there was no room for even a straight pin! But... we were off to the Hall of Fame!

We arrived at Walker's home and began unpacking the car! How in the world did we get all of that in there! We had left early on Friday morning, since I am off work on Fridays. We were a bit tired upon arrival at Walker's, but we all went to Logan's Roadhouse to get a bite to eat because son Kevin works there! He was glad to see all of us! Walker and Sherry joined us and we all had a great time.

Saturday morning we all got up and had our coffee and began to assess the situation on how to arrange everything for the party. We placed a few things here and there and Sherry Mac borrowed the Iron tree for the medals from a florist friend of hers so she and Walker had to go get that and bring it in Walker's van. We had told Sherry there was no budget for decorations, so we just had to be creative with what we had. She had come up with the idea of the tree!

The rest of Saturday and Sunday were taken up with breakfasts, lunches, and visits with friends and family members and a little shopping at Cracker Barrel. John's sister Billie's daughter, Tamara, from California was there and we were happy to see her and visit. The weekend went by fast!

Monday came and we were all working during the day on more things in preparation for the Open House the next night. Soon, it was time to get cleaned up and dressed for the banquet.

Everyone looked great in their banquet clothes and so we all piled into the car and off we went. Upon arriving, and being Christmas, we enjoyed all of the exquisite decorations in the hotel lobby, including a huge tree right in the center, decorated to the max. John had to go check in with the Hall of Fame staff, so the rest of our party made their way downstairs to the open bar for a glass of wine while waiting for the doors to be opened for the banquet. We saw so many family members and friends who had come to celebrate with us. What a time in our life!

The doors were opened and all went in and took their seats. John Jr, Kevin, David McCollum (stepson), Irby McCollum (step grandson), Jo Lowery, sister and Walker, brother and Sherry Mac and I, were all seated together at one table. Jimmy Lowery, Jo's son and his son Reed, were at the same table. All of the others were at two other tables in the large ballroom of about 500 people. John sat on the stage with the other inductees.

Once the dinner was almost finished, they began the program and each inductee walked to the center of the stage, was awarded their plaque, and they then walked out on a runway to have a picture made all while the ~~dossier~~ about them was being read by the Master of Ceremonies. When it was John's turn, all of our tables and some others stood up and cheered and clapped. John felt so good! Nobody in his family has had an honor like this and he is so proud.

When the main event was over and we left our tables, the family and friends gathered over to one side of the ballroom and took pictures and visited with each other. Finally, it was time to go home to Walker's house. Son David and his son Irby had to get back to Arkansas because of their jobs, so would have to miss the open house the next day. By then, we were all pretty tired and ready to relax. We got home and had more wine and finally all went to bed. Tomorrow would be a really busy day for us all.

Tuesday morning we were up early, having our coffee and working on everything from food to re-arranging some furniture etc. Sister Billie had been quite ill and had to come in a wheelchair, so we had to make room to get her in on the first floor dining room.

Iris was just getting her coffee and deciding what she should do next. Cindy was busy helping with doing things like staging the awards on the window sill. Sherry Mac had brought some beautiful rose red brocade fabric and we got a bunch of books and draped them with the fabric in order to elevate some of the pictures and awards. Cindy is great at doing this and when it was done, we placed some votive candles around in between some of the folds of the fabric and it really looked nice. Sherry Mac made a beautiful red, white and blue flower arrangement in a tall crystal vase that sat right behind where the Hall of Fame plaque will be placed.

Iris decorated the cake table with a wonderful picture of John, in a gold frame, placed on a beautiful brass easel. In the picture, he was wearing his running attire, with his three national medals around his neck. She had brought special candlesticks and had red candles in them. We had gotten white napkins printed in gold with "Congratulations John, Hall of Fame 2012". These were on the table with cake plates and utensils. A beautiful gold tablecloth with a red topper, was on the table and the cake was magnificent! It was a huge rectangular cake with white icing and blue trim with little American flags all around the edges standing up on toothpicks. The center of the cake read "Congratulations John, Hall of Fame 2012" and there were large blue stars in a couple of the corners. Sherry Mac had made another beautiful arrangement for the cake table as well as the center of the main food table, all of red, white and blue flowers with red berries and greenery. A silver tier with plates also held chocolate chip cookies beside the cake for desert.

The main food table turned out to be spectacular. Rhonda had brought several elevated dishes so we could get more variety of foods on the main table. We had food galore! Janis made the most wonderful pimento sandwiches on croissants, Rhonda made a hot spinach dip with chips and a chicken salad for another kind of sandwich that was divine. We had salsa with chips, red and green grapes, and a multitude of different cheeses and crackers. There were colorful pinwheel sandwiches that Cindy made that morning while she and Iris were working on the sausages.

I had brought my silver punch bowl and ladle for champagne punch and there was a cranberry punch for those who preferred something plain. These were placed on a lovely wheeled glass cart with cups for serving in the dining room.

In the kitchen, a small table was covered with a plaid tablecloth and had the silver chaffing dish with the sausages in sauce. There was also a big vegetable tray with dip beside the sausages and plates and napkins for those. A smaller flower arrangement enhanced that table too. All around the living room, we had placed smaller bowls of nuts and cheese and cracker plates so anywhere someone sat or stood, they could reach something good to eat.

We were just about ready to get ourselves ready to open the doors and greet our guests! The time had arrived and all of us looked great in our holiday attire!

The guests began arriving and in the kitchen area people were drinking wine and talking and enjoying themselves. So many people came, from family members who had attended the banquet the night before, as well as old friends from way back and some we just had not seen in a very long time. People were looking at the awards and the medal tree and enjoying the food on the main table and visiting with each other down in the dining room. Friends and family members were in the living room visiting with Billie. She was holding up pretty well. Her health had been deteriorating and we were so happy she was able to be there.

Soon, it was time to cut the cake, so everyone came down into the dining room. Sherry Mac broke into song with "He's a Jolly Good Fellow" and everyone else chimed in! There were laughs and clapping and hugs and a few tears too. Pictures were made with Iris at the cake table and Sherry by the tree and Rhonda by the food table, John and Sandy together, and many others with family and friends. The cake was cut and served and it was so yummy!

Everyone really seemed to enjoy themselves and John had a ball! It was a weekday evening because the banquet was planned on Monday, so we had to have the open house on Tuesday, so many had to leave to go to work the next day and some had to get to bed, but all in all, it was a huge success.

Son Kevin, and his friend Rhonda, (see we have two Rhondas and two Sherrys in this family) and John Jr. helped us clean up all that we could that night. Iris, Cindy and I sat down and had a glass of wine before going to bed. We were beat! John Jr.

was leaving early the next day, so he went on to bed. Walker and John and I decided we would go to bed too.

Wednesday morning came all too early for all of us. The girls were recovering from the night before and came in the kitchen for coffee. We started repacking the car and continued cleaning up Walker's house. We had to leave all of the dishes (now clean) for Rhonda, and Walker took the tree back to the florist. Finally, we were ready to go, but it was around 10:00 am or so and we still had a long trip back to Florida ahead of us. We said our goodbyes and thank-yous to Walker and climbed back into the car and headed for home. What an amazing journey!

John here again. Perhaps the best part of this story is all the people who came to share it with me: My bride Sandy; my three boys David (with grandson Irby), John and Kevin; my sisters Jo and Billie; my brother Walker; and other relatives and friends, some of whom I hadn't seen in many years.

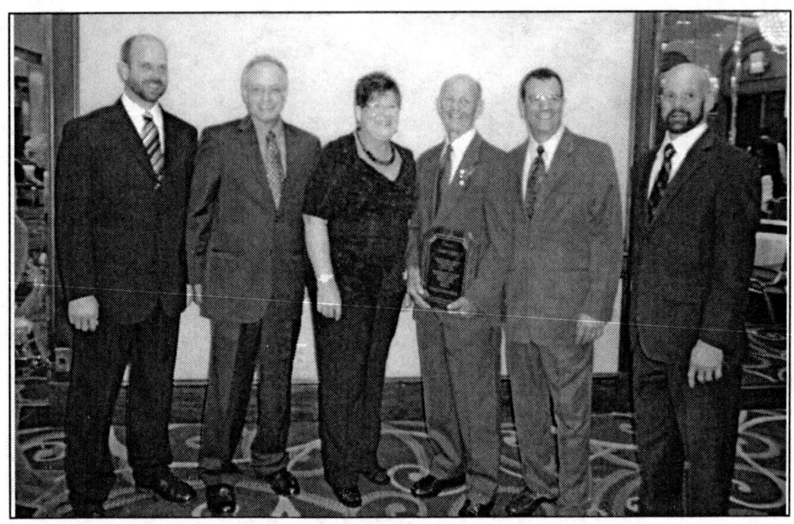

At the Memphis Hall of Fame award banquet, December 3, 2012. L to R: Irby McCollum, his father David McCollum, (my stepson), Sandy and John Hurd, John Hurd Jr. and Kevin Hurd (my two other sons).

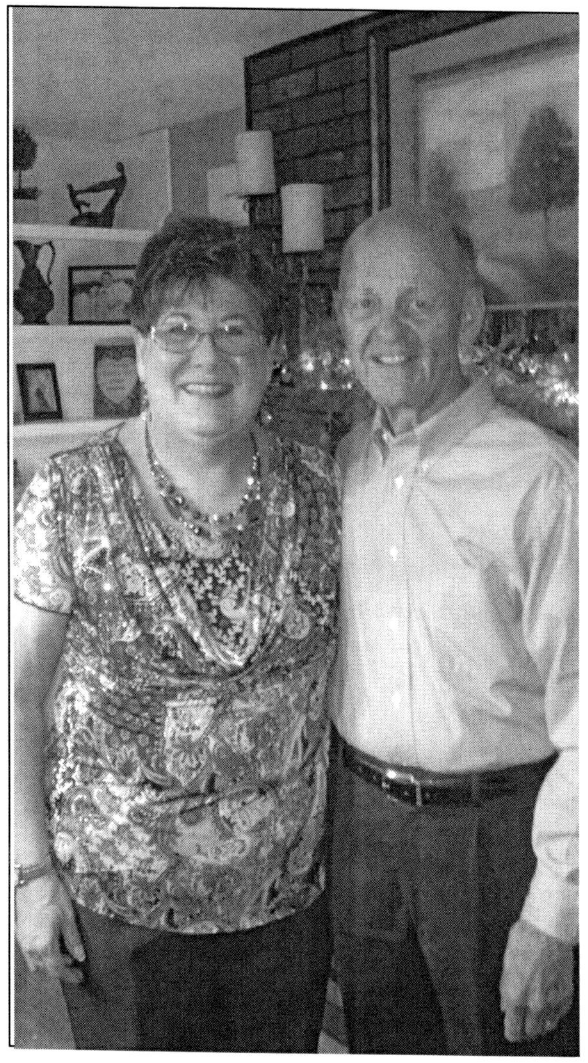

Sandy, my bride of 34 years, and me at the Hall of Fame open house at Walker Hurd's house in 2012.

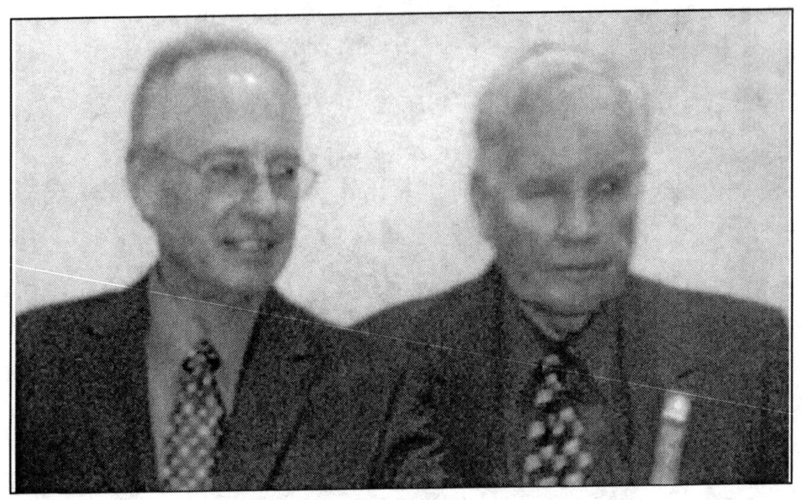

Alex McCollum (right), who sponsored me in the Hall of Fame, with "our" son David McCollum at the Memphis Amateur Sports Hall of Fame award ceremony in 2012.

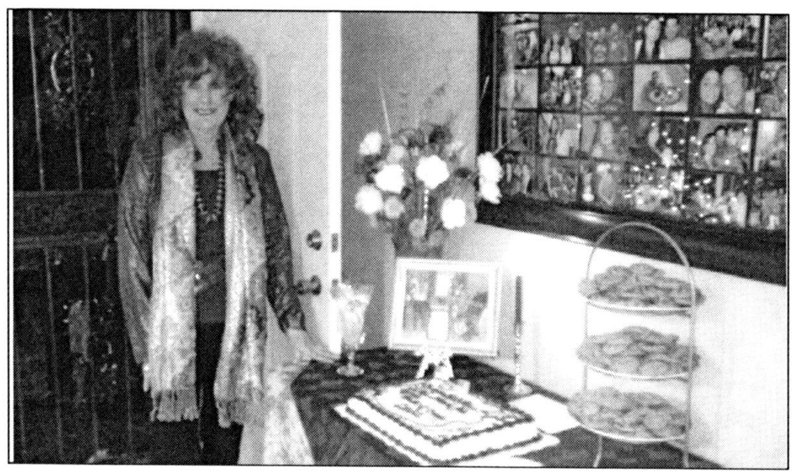

Iris Lawrence, who provided the cake and assisted in preparations for the open house at my brother Walker's house the night after the Hall of Fame awards banquet.

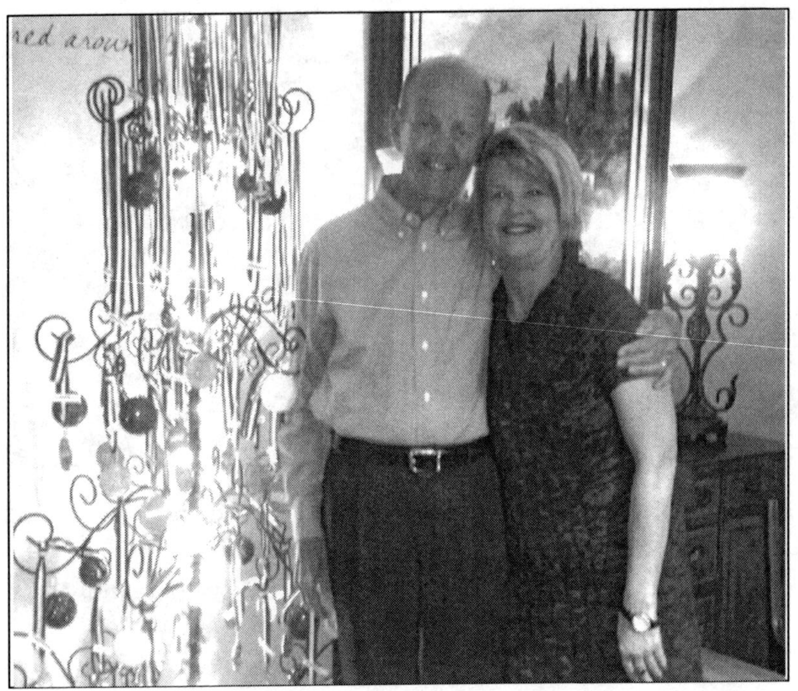

Sherry McClure and the “metal tree of medals” that she created for the open house at Walker’s house the night after the Hall of Fame awards banquet.

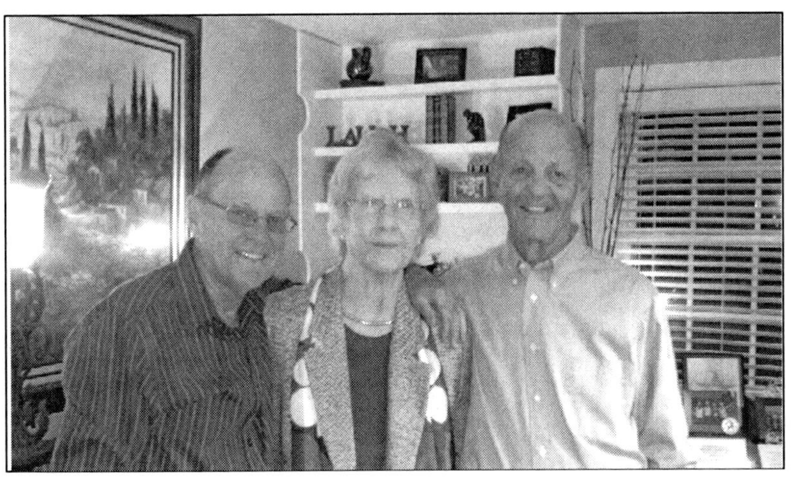

Walker (left) with me and Marian Jernigan, widow of Gene Jernigan, my oldest (since age 4) friend. Walker and I considered Gene to be our brother, which makes Marian our sister-in-law.

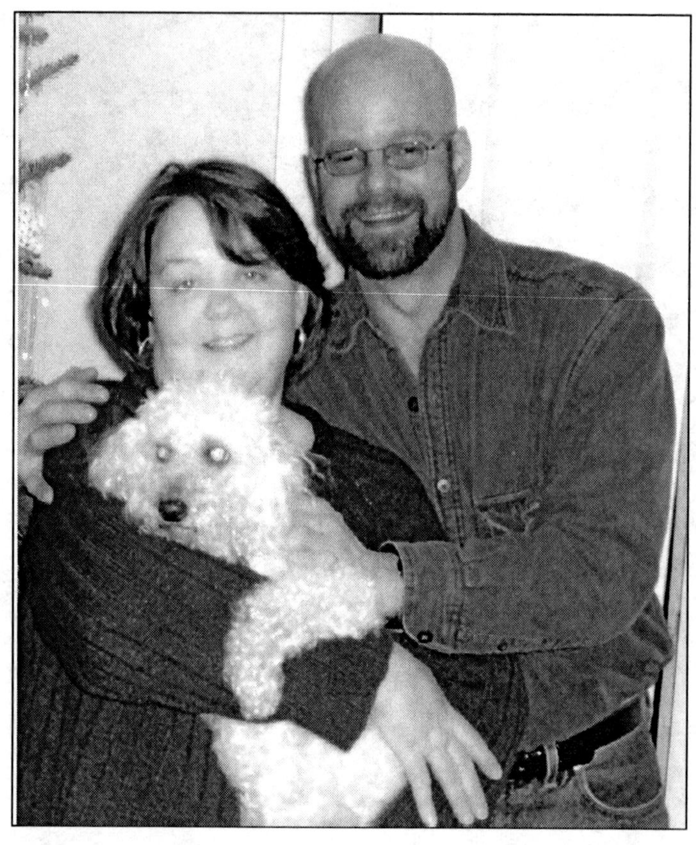

My son, Kevin Hurd and his friend and neighbor Rhonda Young.

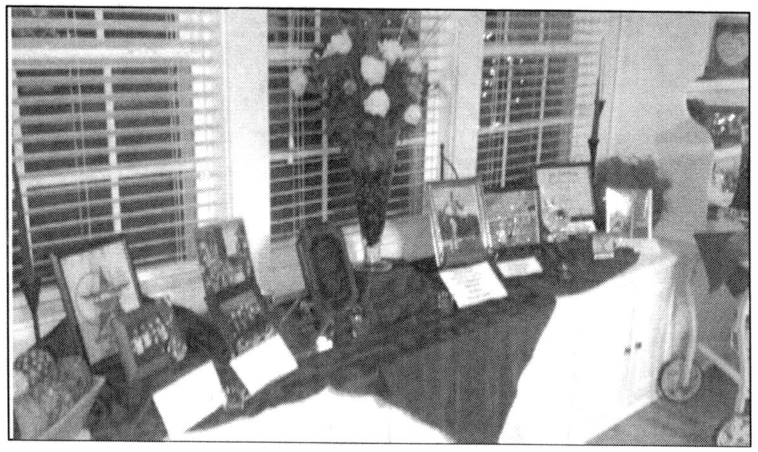

The "Award Stage" at the open house at brother Walker's house the night after the Hall of Fame banquet.

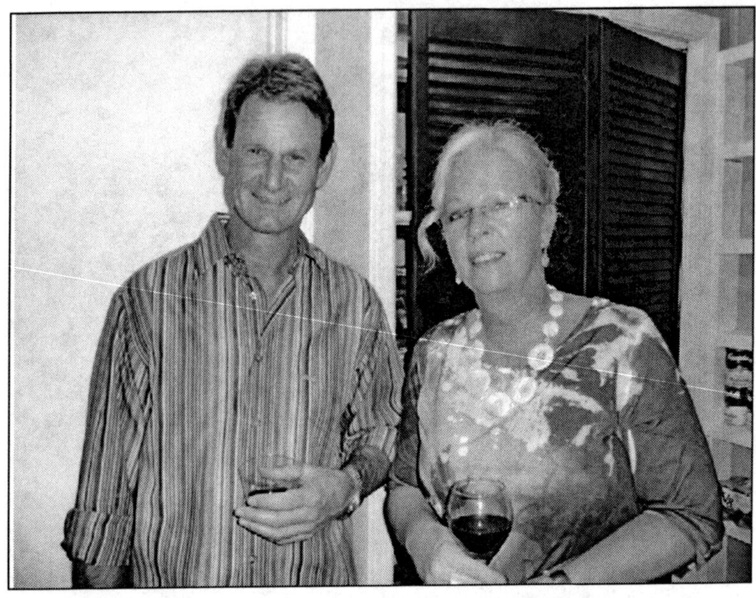

Jimmy Lowery (Jo's son), helped with the food, and Cindy Hibbard, who was chief architect in staging of the awards at the open house.

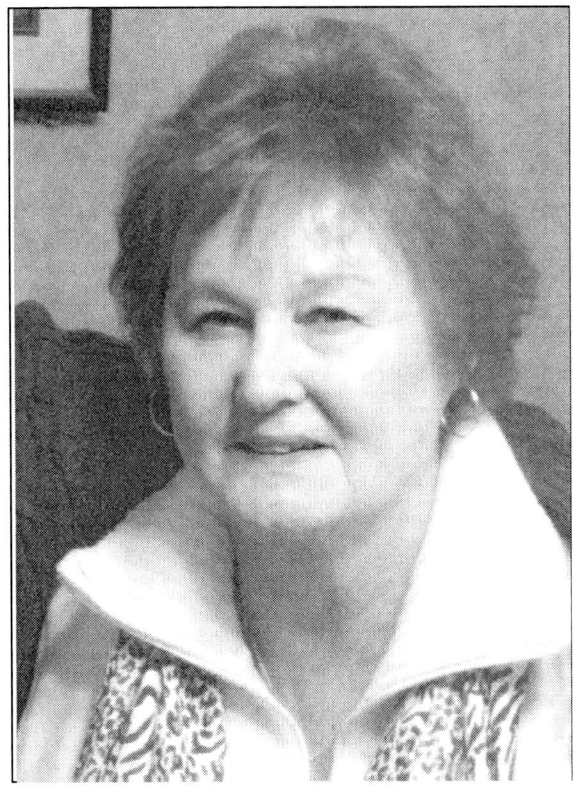

Jo's daughter, Susan Lewis, helped prepare for the open house at Walker's house.

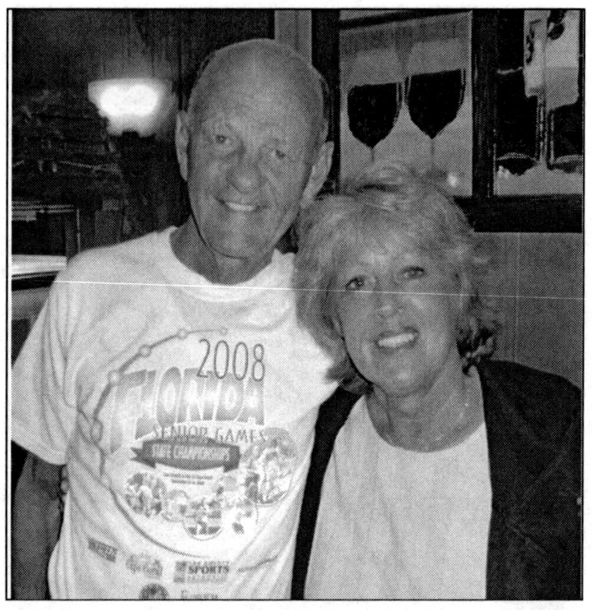

John and Sherry Campbell, Jo's daughter, one of the worker "elves" at the party.

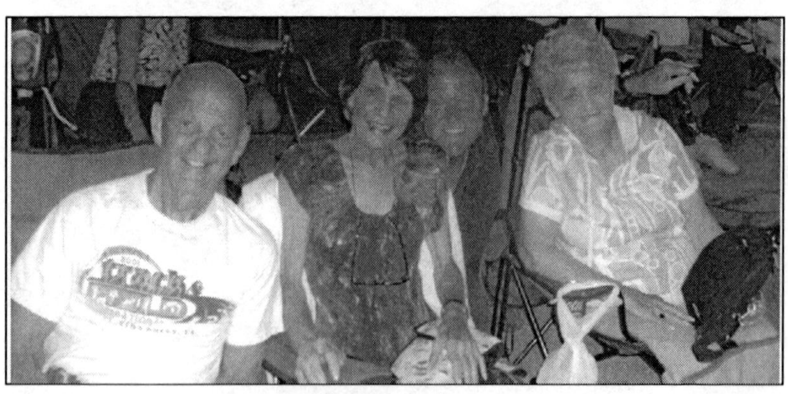

Four of the five original Hurd siblings: L to R John, Billie, Walker, Jo

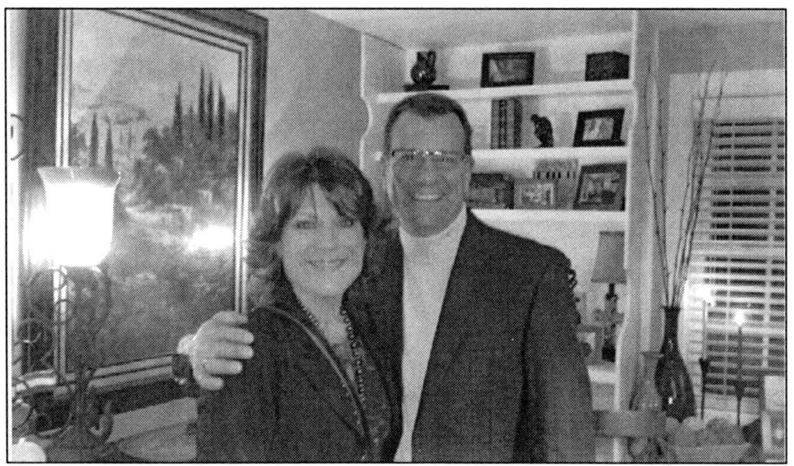

Walker's daughter Janis with my son John Jr., who drove in from Baltimore to help with the party.

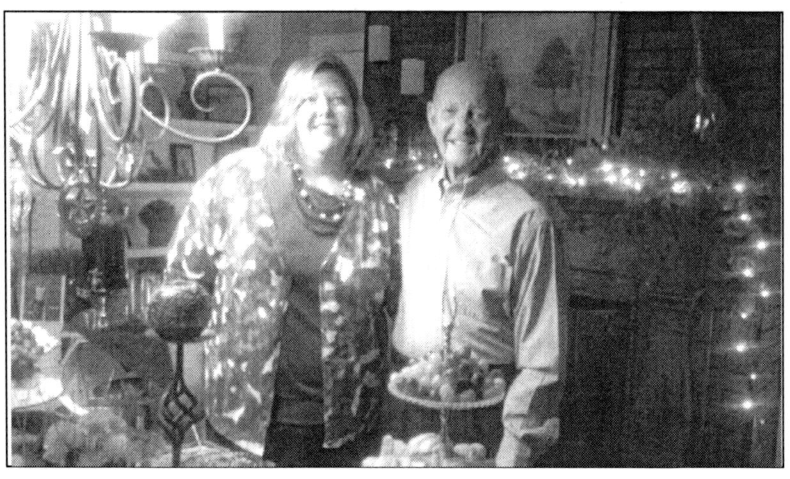

Rhonda Hurd, Walker's daughter-in-law, with me, and some of the food she helped with for the party.

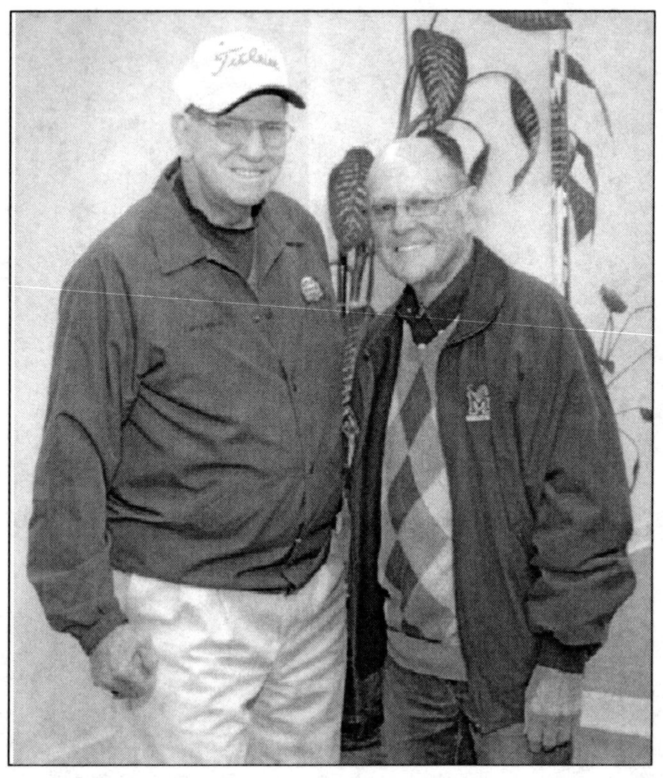

Larry Hilbun who, with Alex McCollum, sponsored and did the ground work for getting me nominated and elected to the Memphis Amateur Sports Hall of Fame in 2012. He's with his golfing buddy, my brother Walker.

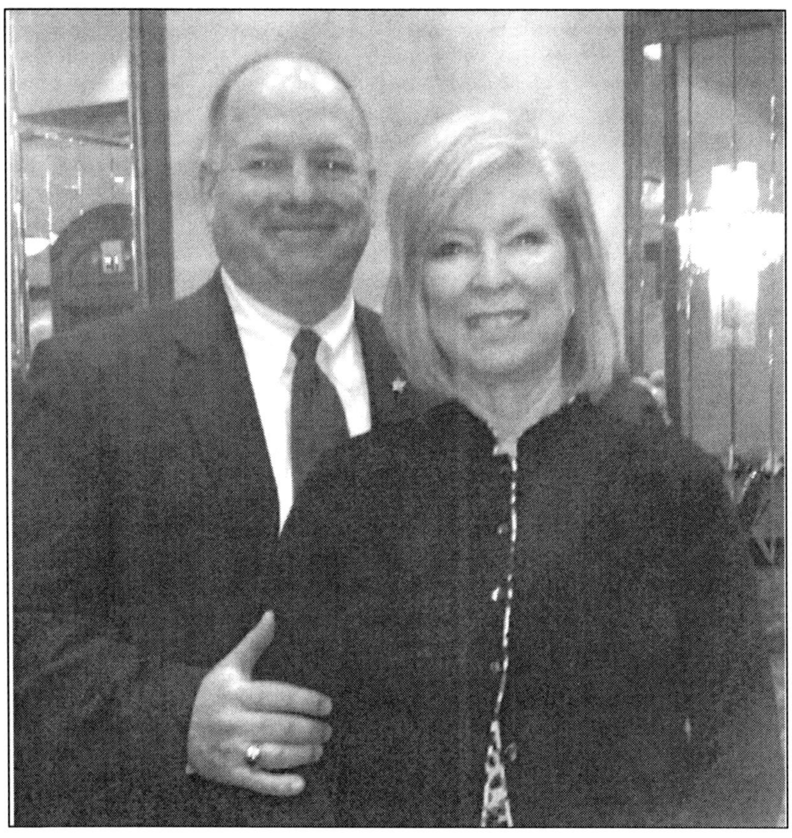

Bert and Rayanna Bailey, our former business associates, drove from Knoxville, TN for the Hall of Fame inductions.

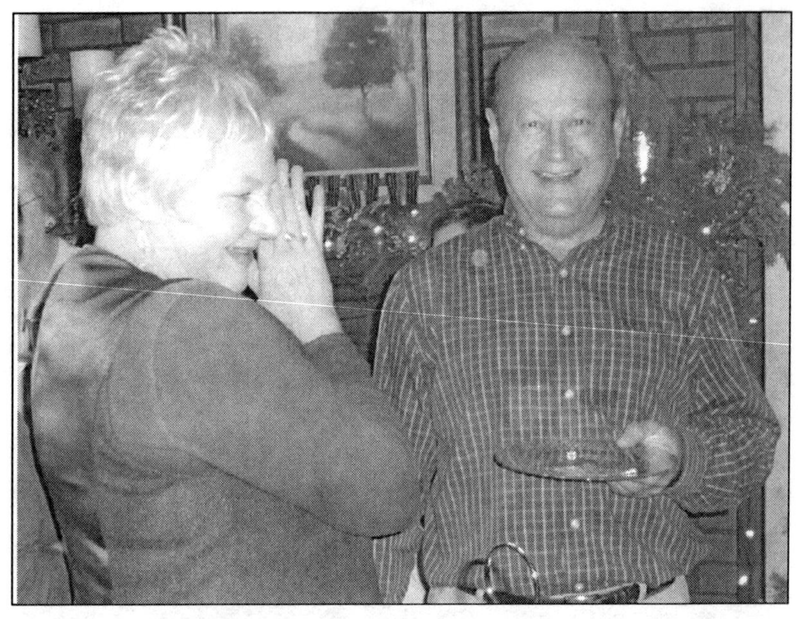

Susan and Jeff Shotwell, my sister Billie's son, at the open house the night after the Hall of Fame inductions.

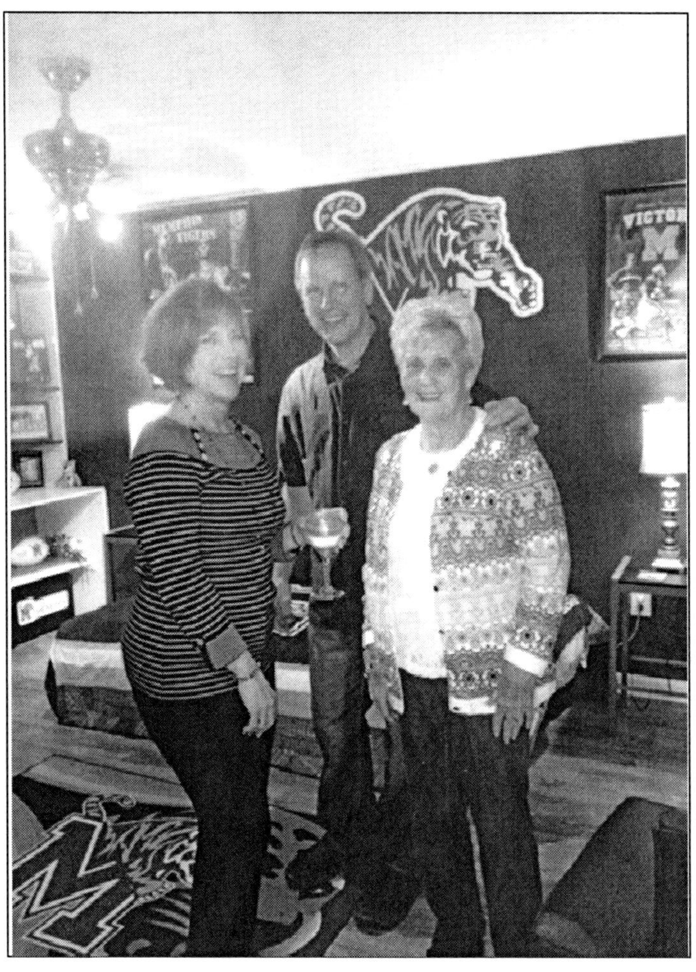

Tamara Ogburn and David McClellan flew in from San Juan Capistrano, CA and from Boise, ID to see their mother, Billie and get her to the open house. With their Aunt Jo in Uncle Walker's Tiger Den (Univ. of Memphis fan).

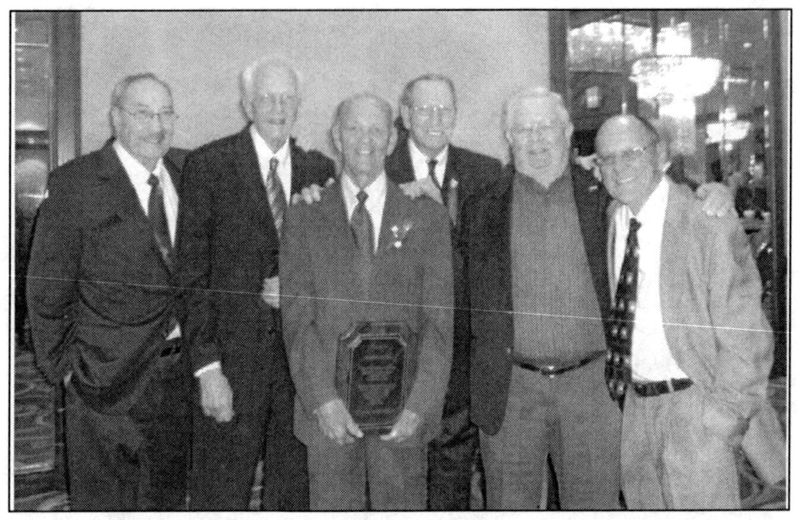

Sigma Phi Epsilon brothers all, at the Hall of Fame induction. L to R Bill Caldwell, Dan Goodwin, John Hurd, Larry Hilbun, Walter Robbins, Walker Hurd.

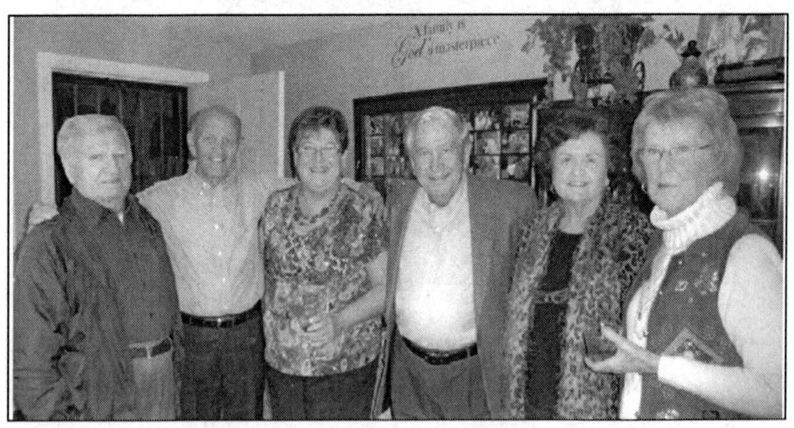

Close friends of 60 plus years after the Hall of Fame induction. L to R Bob White, John and Sandy Hurd, Lou and Frances Ricossa, and Wilda White, Bob's wife.

19
The Dream is Real

Well, we drove the 500 miles home from the Memphis festivities on Wednesday, I unpacked and repacked on Thursday, drove 475 miles to Winter Haven, Florida on Friday the 7th, and the year 2012 ended with a hat trick at the Florida Games on Sunday the 9th. For the first time, the 50 meter dash became an official event in Florida. I won the gold medal with a World Class time of 8.90 seconds. I also won the gold in both the 100m and 200m dashes, making it 10 years in a row for both of those events. The times were both All American, 16.56 and 35.00 seconds respectively.

As a warm-up for the Nationals in 2013, I competed in the Mississippi Games in Clinton in June, winning the 50m in 7.97 (World Class), the 100m in 16.19 (All American), and the 200m in 35.41 (All American). Phil and Cathy Campbell were not present this time.

Then it started to get exciting. My youngest son, Kevin, called me from Memphis and asked about motel availability and rates in Cleveland. I asked "Are you thinking about coming to the National Championships?" He was! He had already arranged to fly in on Tuesday, July 23rd, and stay for the whole show! I assured him that his room was paid for, because mine had two beds, and was conveniently located between the airport and the track at Baldwin Wallace University, which actually is in Berea, Ohio.

On the day before I was to leave for Cleveland, I received a call from Nick Gandy, Director of Communications at the Florida Sports Authority. He had been reviewing some statistics and noticed that I had won both of the dashes 10 out of 10 years. He has a friend with the *Pensacola News Journal*, and had called him to tell him about me and what was coming up. He said I would probably get a call from him, and "hoped I didn't mind." Duh! Does a bear mind if you give him honey?

The drive to Cleveland was two and a half days, stopping over in Decatur, AL and Columbus, OH. I checked in on Monday and went to the track for a light workout. Tuesday I rested, then met Kevin's delayed plane at 8 pm.

Now I had a decision to make. I had been starting my races from a standing position for years, wanting to be sure that the blood flow would get to my brain ok. If I'm going to run my best, in an all-out effort to win, I've got to suck it up and use the three point start that Phil Campbell showed me on his DVD. If coming up off of ground level suddenly at top speed was going to be a problem, then so be it, but I had to give it a go.

The first event Wednesday was the 100 meter prelim at 8 am. John Wall and I were in the same heat, and both of us qualified for the finals. That afternoon we ran the 200m prelims. John did not show up for that one, but I again qualified for the finals. I think John and his lady friend, Dora Yates, were sightseeing.

Thursday was another special day for me. I was expecting two of our friends from the Core Living gatherings in Michigan to drive over from their Ohio homes, two and three hours away. Warming up for the 50m prelims at 11 am, I looked over at the stands, and there they were: Susan Romanski and Carolyn Weislogel. They had known Kevin would be there, had already identified him (probably from our family resemblance and matching no-hairdos), and they were all seated together. Wow! My very own groupies.

The top three times in the 50m prelims were mine at 8.72, Ron Gray from Colorado at 8.98, and John Wall at 9.19. I mention that here because when we ran the finals the next day, we again finished in that order, but the clock did not activate with the starter gun's firing, so we had no times. All we knew was who won which medal. As I described in Chapter 7, they later used our prelim times as finals. Since that was the first time for the 50m dash in the National Games, my 8.72 seconds is a new record.

At 4 pm the same day, we ran the 100m finals. I placed first in 16.16 seconds, All American and World Class (and better than I had done two years earlier in Humble, Texas), followed by Ronald Gray at 16.75, Alexander Johnson from New Jersey at 17.21, and John Wall at 17.64, and others. All of the first four earned All American honors. It was my first individual gold medal at the national level, and one of my boys and two friends were there to witness it. As we used to say in west Tennessee, "It can't hardly git no better'n that."

Later that day, we were all gathered around for the presentation of medals. After more than an hour I began to get hungry. I started moaning about how long this was taking, can't they get on with it, etc. Putting it all into perspective, Kevin leaned over to me and said "Dad, you've waited 20 years for this, your first individual national level gold medal. Surely you can wait 20 more minutes." Ouch.

The next morning was Friday, the last day of track events. At 8:35 we ran the 50m, and as you already know, the top three were me, followed by Ronald Gray and John Wall, with unknown times because of the failure of the clock.

At 10:35 am we ran the 200m. Again, the top four all ran All American times. I placed 1st with 35.66 seconds, 2nd was Alexander Johnson (NJ) at 37.38, 3rd was Halbert Goolsby (VA), my high school friend at 37.94, and 4th was Tom Jenkins (OH) at 38.67. Six events down, one to go.

The 4x100 meter relay got off at 4:10 pm. By the way, of all eight of the National events I have participated in, this was probably the best organized with respect to sticking to a schedule. Usually they will list a starting time for a particular activity, then with luck it starts on time. In Cleveland they listed the times, itemized by age groups, and you'd darn well better be there ready to go at that time. Kudos to all of them for organizing and executing plans and schedules as well as they did. It is a tremendous job and my hat is off to all of them.

Charlie Baker, John Wall and I were the three who had been there for all three of the "Tennessee" relay teams (2007, 2011, and 2013). This time we were fortunate in being able to recruit another Tennessee boy, Halbert Goolsby, my high school classmate who now resides in Virginia. Our running order was: Baker, Goolsby, Wall and Hurd. We won with a new American record time of 1:15.99 (one minute and 15.99 seconds), ahead of the number two team who registered a time of 1:28.58, a difference of about 55 meters or 60 yards.

The decision to use the new starting position was the correct one. I know it made a difference in my performance. Thanks, Phil and Cathy Campbell.

I was one spent young man after those three days, but I had a feeling of euphoria unlike almost anything I had ever felt before. I had trained and competed every week for 20 years, not always as diligently as I should have, and certainly not always patiently, but with the dream that eventually I would get the brass ring. And I took home four of them from Cleveland. To have two friends take their entire day off to drive the miles and be there for that most meaningful day, and to have one of my three sons there to share every minute of the 72 hours with me, was an extra special blessing that I could have only hoped for. Thanks, Goomba, for helping your old man to celebrate three of the best days of my life (the small percentage of it that I have experienced so far).

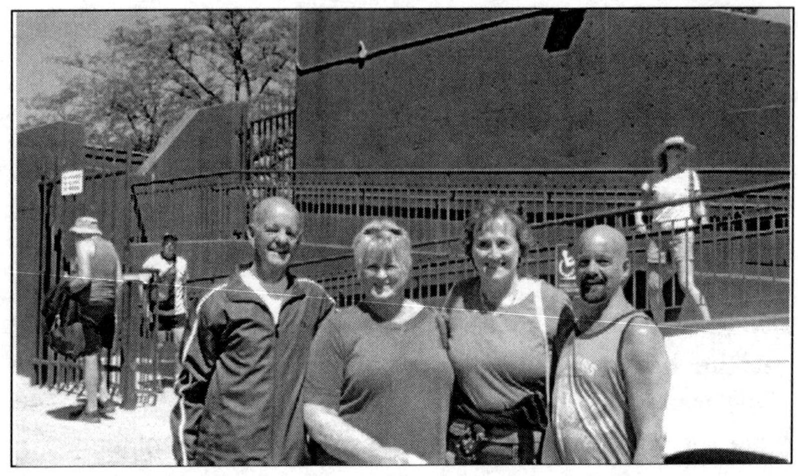

My "Groupies" at the Senior Games National Championships in Cleveland, Ohio July 25, 2013.

L to R John Hurd, Susan Romanski, Carolyn Weislogel, and my son Kevin Hurd. Susan and Carolyn drove in for the day from their Ohio homes two and three hours away. Kevin flew in from Memphis, Tennessee to spend the entire three days with me.

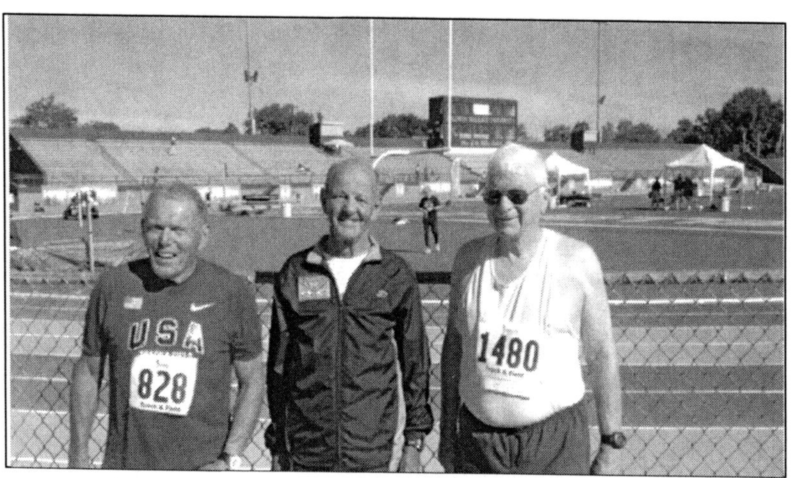

The top three winners of the Men's age 80-84 50 meter dash, 2013 Senior Games National Championships in Cleveland, Ohio. Left to right: Ron Gray 2nd, John Hurd 1st, John Wall 3rd.

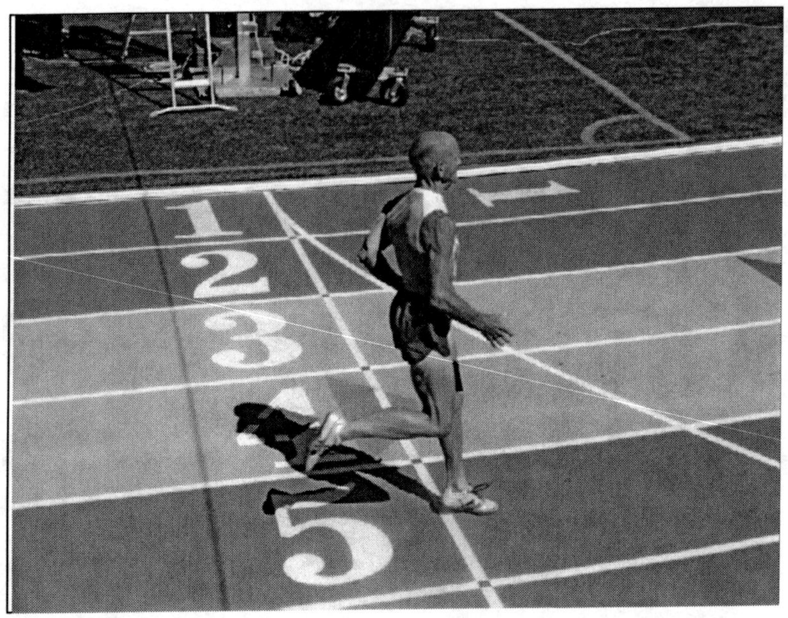

My first individual gold medal at the national level – the age 80-84 100 meter dash at the Senior Games National Championships in Cleveland, Ohio July 25, 2013. Time 16.16 seconds. Photo by Rhonda Young and Kevin Hurd.

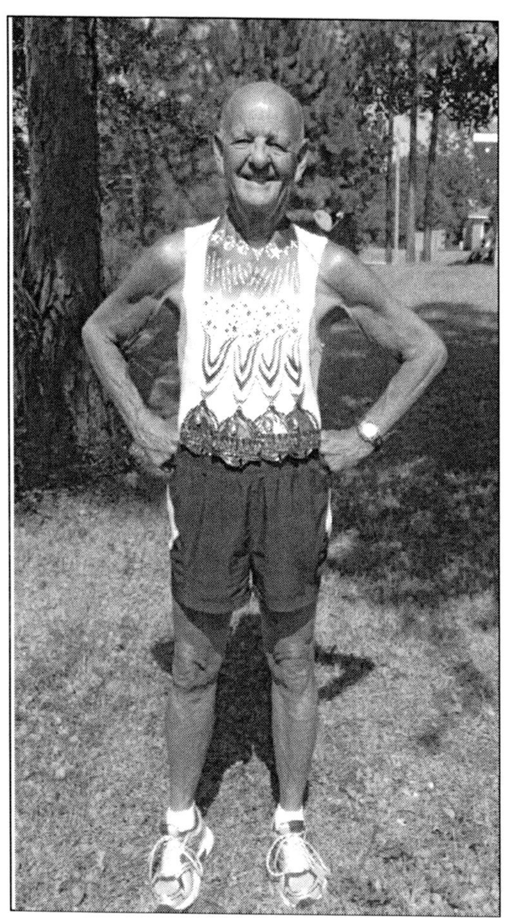

And here they are, four medals for the 50, 100, and 200 meter dashes and the 4x100 meter relay.

20
Another Hurd Heard From

Note: *Since this was the first opportunity any of my boys had had to experience the major games with me, Sandy thought it would be good to invite Kevin to share his thoughts on the Cleveland National Championships. He agreed, and I promised him I wouldn't change a word, and that I would not show him my text beforehand. Here, then, are Kevin's thoughts on the games, and his father in general.*

I think the wheels started turning in my head when Dad first mentioned that the National Senior Games were coming up soon, and that he was going to Cleveland to compete. Although at this point he had won enough state titles in the 50 meter, 100 meter, and 200 meter races to remind me of Lucy Van Pelt trying to count raindrops (he had enough medals and ribbons to decorate a pretty good-sized Christmas tree), I had only seen him run once, and that was at a local meet. He had also never won an individual gold in the National games, and I couldn't shake the feeling that this time he was going to take home the prize.

The more I thought about it, the more I became convinced that if I blew this opportunity to see him run in a title tilt (yes, I know that's a boxing term), I might never get another chance. Sure, I could catch him winning another state meet, but those had become routine – if he ran, he won. The medals that meant the most to him were the two silvers he had won in the previous national games (in the 100 and 200 meter heats), and I knew he was going to be gunning for the gold this time. I also knew that he might or might not compete the next time the nationals were held, so the time to go see him was now. I kept thinking that if I missed seeing him winning the national gold when I could have gone, I would never forgive myself.

I wasn't really sure if he would even want me to go. I didn't think Sandy usually went to his meets, and I wondered if my presence might throw him off his game, or worse, jinx him. So, instead of just calling him up and saying, "Hi, Dad, I'm coming to Cleveland to watch you run – which way to the stadium?" I called to ask him about hotel prices in the area. When he suggested that I just room with him, I knew he was not only okay with my coming, but actually liked the idea. At that point it was on.

After doing a little math, I decided that flying wasn't a whole lot more expensive than driving, and it would be a heckuva lot more fun. I hadn't flown in years, and that would make the trip even more enjoyable. Dad had gotten over the excitement of flying before I was even born, I think, because he had made so many trips while working for IBM back in the day. He had also been lucky enough to miss a flight or two that had wound up crashing. If I remember right, he believed that Braniff Airlines was a pack full of death traps.

At the time that I made the flight reservations, Dad wasn't really expecting to run in the 4x100 meter relay, but I knew that if I scheduled an early flight out, the opportunity to run in that event would present itself - Murphy's law being what it is – and Dad would be stuck with having to take me to the airport when he could have been competing. He and his partners had won the gold twice before in the National games, and I figured that the relay was a guaranteed victory with which to end the week. I couldn't let him miss that, so I scheduled the later departure. This turned out to be a wise move.

Just hanging out with my dad over the next few days was half the fun of the trip. This was the first time in a very long time that we had had time to just sit and talk. Now, this did involve going to bed early and getting up early (two things to which I was decidedly unaccustomed), but it was well worth it. One of the stories he told me during that week was the one about dancing onstage with the bottoms of his feet torn off – I had never heard that one before, and it was pretty hilarious. I won't go into detail on it because I'm pretty sure he covers it elsewhere in this book. As good as Dad is at telling a story on paper, he's even better live, because he's a natural actor. He could probably make a story about drying socks sound interesting.

Dad's offbeat sense of humor is never far from the surface. I am told (and I'll bet it's true) that on the day I was born, he said to Mom - who had been hoping for a girl – "Well, honey, it's a boy. Should we throw him back?" I'm sure Mom knew he was kidding, but she probably gave him hell for it anyway, just on general principle.

Dad's the sort of fellow who, when the telephone rings, is liable to deadpan "Better answer that – it might be a phone call." When my brothers and I were kids, we learned not to ask for something by saying "Can I?" If one of us asked Dad, "Can I go outside and play?" Dad would reply "I don't know – are you able? Your legs look like they work fine to me. I would assume that you're able – maybe you had a different question in mind."

The point, of course, was that the request was properly made with a "may I" rather than a "can I." Today I have a degree in English, but if Dad catches me on a point of grammar, I automatically know he's right – I don't have to bother looking it up in my Strunk and White. (By the way, I realized several years too late that the proper response to the "may I/can I" correction would have been to ask him "May I do such and such?" and after he replied, "Yes, you may", to zing him with "Then again, I may not!")

Once, when a friend of mine and I were trying to cook up a good non sequitur riddle, we had come up with the following: "If you're digging a semicircular jelly canal with a piece of guardrail stolen from the living room of the Taj Mahal by half a dozen paranoid pygmies wearing combat Bermuda shorts, how many..." – and there we were stuck. It occurred to me that this was the sort of thing Dad would be a natural at, so we decided to ask him for some ideas. Without missing a beat, he answered, "How many hummingbirds with chapped lips does it take to pluck all the pimientos out of a jar of olives?" Our search was over, just like that. If you're curious about the answer to the riddle, it's pi – because early fourteenth century Japanese fighter buses had foam rubber U-joints to facilitate hexagonal conversation.

Much of this book is of course concerned with Dad's running career, but his emergence as the fastest octogenarian in the country was a fairly late development. Among other things, he had to wait the required eighty years to reach octogenarian status. On the other hand, he has always been the smartest person I know for any age – his mind works even faster than his legs. Dad can rattle off the value of the aforementioned pi to a couple of dozen decimal places, remembers license plate numbers that he saw fifty years ago (along with the make and model of the car and the exact date on which he saw it), can tell you what day of the week you were born on if you tell him the date, and handily whipped both me and my mother at a game that requires one to quickly come up with as many words as one can from a group of letters. Mom and I prided ourselves on our skills at those types of games – not without reason – but Dad flat out dogged us in game after game one night, and we were forced to admit that we had more than met our match. It hardly seemed fair – we both knew he was a math whiz, but we thought we had a fighting chance in a game of words. Dad sees patterns quickly, remembers details forever, and explains points of logic in terms that can be understood. That's part of what makes him a natural teacher.

I have no doubt that one of the reasons Dad's mind has stayed so sharp over the years is the running. There's nothing like good hard exercise and focusing on a goal to keep the body and mind both healthy and in well-oiled working condition. It also gets him compliments from the girls – I've heard more than one woman my age or younger saying "Hey – your Dad's got nice legs". I myself have the sort of legs that only a bird could love (although I do have a pretty cool scar left over from my little league days). That permanent tan he gets from running in the Florida sun doesn't hurt, either.

The success Dad had once he started getting really serious about his running didn't really surprise me, as I recall. He's the sort of person whom one expects to do well at any task he decides to take on. If he decides that he is going to write a program to perform a certain difficult task on a computer, I have no doubt that he'll get that program done and that it will be more concise and more efficient than whatever the next fellow could come up with. Running was just a different task, but the results were the same.

For years I had heard about his success on the track and seen the medals that he accumulated, but I had never seen him actually run in a big race. I knew that once he got rolling he took home the gold in the Tennessee state championships every year, and when he moved to Florida, he did the same thing. I guess I just sort of took it for granted the way I took his status as a Professor Emeritus for granted. Hey, that was my dad – he's supposed to be the smartest, and if he runs, then he's supposed to be the fastest. For one thing Dad loves numbers, and sprinting is all about numbers. Dad kept precise track of his progress in his times in the various sprints, and knew exactly what he needed to gain All-America status, world class status, and what the best times were for his upcoming opponents. I really think for him this was a big part of the fun. He could calculate the exact time that he would need to achieve whatever his next goal was, and then enjoy the process of watching his numbers improve until he met that goal.

I think another big part of the fun Dad was having during those years was all the people he met. When he talked about his upcoming races, he referred to his opponents by their first names. They weren't just the guys against whom he was running – they were friends. These folks in the senior games don't just go out there and silently compete against one another – they get to know each other. It's a very friendly sport, I believe, and that's quite understandable. After all, these athletes are doing something most people their ages don't do – they run outside and play! Don't they know they're supposed to be sitting on a couch exercising their thumbs on the remote? I would think that it makes for a natural sense of camaraderie among them to be doing something that not too many people are doing. It is probably not unlike the bond that players feel in a chess club, or that amateur astronomers feel when they get together to roam among the stars with their telescopes. It's the very pleasant feeling of knowing that one is surrounded by people with the same interests and the same drive as oneself. And unlike the sedentary activities of chess and stargazing, these people are doing something that gives them an energy that few people in general, and even fewer over fifty, get in their daily lives. Quite frankly, I envy that!

I'm one of those people who can't use coffee to get their energy because even one or two cups makes my hair stand on end. Fortunately, the hotel where we were staying served free decaf, and the hot beverage along with the various flavors they offered were enough to wake me up for those early mornings without bugging my eyes out. Dad's first prelim was for the 100 meter dash on Wednesday morning at the ungodly hour of nine o'clock (the sun was still shaving), and he knocked it down with a first place finish. Since he had never won an individual medal in the national games before, that was a great way to kick things off. When the afternoon rolled around and he placed second in the 200 meter prelim, things were looking good for the home team.

The next morning's 50 meter prelim was held at the much more reasonable hour of eleven, and Dad had the best time. With all three of the qualifying runs finished, I was projecting two golds and a silver for him, and had already decided that my decision to come to Cleveland for these games showed excellent timing on my part. It was clear to me by this point that I was going to be the first family member to witness Dad winning national medals, and that he was likely to get one in all three events. In the meantime, I was still trying to figure out the best way to get pictures using my phone, Dad's phone, and my friend Rhonda's camera. One thing I had decided on – I would position myself right at the finish line. If indeed one or more of the races wound up in a photo finish, I wanted to see for myself who was ahead when the line was crossed.

The first race for all the marbles was in the latter part of the afternoon, so we had plenty of time to grab some lunch and rest up for what was to me the main event – the 100 meter dash. The 50 meter, 200 meter, and relay are all great, but the 100 is the classic event. I suppose that if he had been trying out for the National Senior Football League, I would have been more concerned about his time in the 40, but this was track. The key would be how quickly I could snap the pictures, so I elected to use Rhonda's camera rather than either of the phones.

This turned out to be another case of excellent timing on my part. The one occasion on which I got a perfect picture on any of the devices was during the race that I wanted most for Dad to win, and I nailed it right as he was crossing the finish line well ahead of the competition. My favorite part of this photo is the detail on Dad's right shoulder. The cording on it makes it look like the muscle is made out of piano wire. It reminds me of Bruce Lee's muscles. This is the picture I showed to everyone at work after I returned from Cleveland to do my bragging tour. First, however, I had to endure a few minutes of panic when I couldn't find the bloody picture on my phone. I finally realized that it would be under downloads rather than photos. I will say that it made a wonderful wallpaper for a while. As a matter of fact, Dad was my wallpaper star for quite some time after the games. I used pictures of him with his new medals, pictures of the medal "tree" he has at home, et cetera, et cetera.

The 50 meter final was another victory for us, but it came with a frustrating problem. This being the first time that the 50 was run in the national games meant that the winner would automatically have the American record. Unfortunately, there was no signal from the pistol to start the clock, which meant that there was no time to record. Dad and some other participants lobbied to have the 8.72 second time logged in the prelim used as the official time, but to no avail. The upshot of all that is that Dad will go down as the first ever winner of the fifty meter dash in the national games, but the next fellow to win it will have the American record. You know, now that I think about it, that's a pretty good incentive for Dad to compete the next time the national games are held!

The 200 meter final was the last of the individual races for him, and this time I made a decision which turned out to be the right one. All during the events I had been trying to capture the moments with well-timed photos, but with the exception of the killer shot of the 100 meter finish, I had struggled. I was also quite frankly getting tired of watching the races through a tiny screen. I hadn't flown all this way to watch everything on a four inch window – I wanted to see the events live. With that in mind, I asked one of the fellows in the stands with me if he wouldn't mind videotaping the 200 meter for me, since he didn't have anyone he knew in the race. He agreed, and I was able to just enjoy watching and cheering this time rather than fiddling with the camera. Bless his heart! It's hard to see the first half of that race because of all the people standing and yelling in front of us, but for the last fifty yards or so, he got a nice clear shot of Dad leaving the field behind, and I made sure practically everyone I knew saw that video.

After that race, we had about seven hours to kill before the 4x100 relay, giving us plenty of time to enjoy the sensation of having, not just a medal or two (which would have been wonderful by itself), but three - and all of them gold! Dad was officially the fastest man in the country his age or older, and he and several of his friends (including, I believe, a fellow he went to high school with – imagine that), had decided to enter the relay with Dad, of course, as the anchor. Since he already had two gold medals from the previous national games in that event, I had no doubt that he would be packing four of those bad boys in his suitcase for the trip back home and still have time to drop me off at the airport, thanks to my sensible decision to take the later flight.

That race turned out to be a blowout – Dad could have played hopscotch for the last hundred meters and still won – but he and his partners ran it full tilt just the same. The result was a new American record, and THIS one had an official time to go with it – 75.99 seconds. It also happened to be the very last event of the games. What a way to end the show. Four events had yielded four gold medals, and Dad had finally accomplished everything there was to accomplish in his chosen field. I have always known that he was the smartest person I've ever met, and one of the very few truly, truly good people I have ever known, but now I can say – and I do – that my Dad is flat out (with apologies to Billy Clyde Puckett) the hummingest sumbitch in America!

John's Note: *In Dan Jenkins's book "Semi-Tough," about a professional football team in Texas, one of the major characters was a colorful player named Billy Clyde Puckett. The last line in the last paragraph above, Kevin quoted from and attributed to Mr. Puckett.*

21
My 15 More Minutes

I arrived home from Cleveland on Saturday, and on Monday I received the anticipated phone call from a sports reporter at the *Pensacola News Journal*. He had heard from Nick Gandy at the Florida Sports Authority and had a lot of questions for me. I met his photographer at a high school track in Pensacola for pictures, and the next Saturday they ran a super story with a giant action picture on page one of the sports section.

On Monday, two days after that story ran, I got another call from the *Northwest Florida Daily News*, the local paper that I subscribe to. They wanted to do a story on me also. (Why did I get the idea that they learned about me from reading the Pensacola paper?) They placed their story and picture on page one as their lead headline for the day. I loved it!

Shortly after that, I got a call from Larry Hilbun in Memphis telling me that Edgar Buffaloe had been nominated for the Memphis Amateur Sports Hall of Fame, by a fellow boxer and former classmate of Edgar, Gordon "Red" Gilbert. Alright!! Edgar's wife, Jean, had sent some background material to them, and I had previously gathered everything I had on him in anticipation, and organized that and sent it in also.

A short time later Larry called me again to tell me that Edgar had been selected unanimously. Another automatic decision was made; I had to go to Memphis for the award ceremony. At this point I must tell you something. Before moving to Panama City Beach, Florida in 2001, Edgar had suffered a stroke which affected his short term memory. After they, and a little later Sandy and I, moved here to Florida he had a head injury, which did not help the situation at all.

We sent our reservation request in, and learned that we would be seated at the table with Edgar's wife, Jean, and Roy, his younger brother.

The night of the banquet and ceremony, we got there early and I took a position near the front door of the hotel to look for Jean and Edgar. The door was all glass and revolving, the perimeter of which was also all glass, with one opening. While watching for the Buffaloes, I noticed two gentlemen in the revolving door, and one of them, thinking he had reached the opening, walked right smack dab in to the glass wall, dropping to the floor on his back. I rushed over to help the other man assist him to his feet and recognized that he was Gordon "Red" Gilbert, the man who had nominated Edgar. I said "You're Gordon Gilbert," and he said "Yeah, I remember you; you were at Memphis State when I was. You know, the best boxers in the Mid-South tried to take me down, but that glass wall was the first one to succeed." We got a Band-Aid put on near his eye and he was in good shape.

I returned to my lookout position and soon Jean and Edgar came in. I greeted him with a bear hug, and we almost got a little emotional, the same as I am doing as I write this. He still remembers me, and the 66 years we've been close friends; he just doesn't remember where I live, or recent events, like when we last saw each other.

All of the inductees were seated on the stage once the meal and ceremonies began. When Edgar's turn came to be honored, he stood there clutching his award proudly, and holding back the emotional expression that I recognized, and perhaps most of the people present did not. I knew that he was aware of where he was and what was happening. I also knew that despite all of that, he would not remember any of it the next day. And Jean confirmed later that he did not.

So, was it all for nothing? No, no, no indeed. I would have gone anywhere in the country to see him live that one moment, relishing the praise and recognition that he so richly deserved. It was worth every bit of it.

The totally unexpected phone call

I had won my events at the Pensacola Games earlier in September, but did not make it to the state finals in Fort Myers after the Hall of Fame trip. It was the first time I had missed a state finals in the 20 years that I had been competing. Sandy had a health situation come up while we were in Memphis for Edgar's celebration, 13 days before the Florida finals, and I stayed home to look after her. After all that she has endured and given up so that I could pursue my hobby, that decision was also automatic. Fortunately, she has recovered remarkably well.

Now it was Thursday, February 20, 2014. I was in Burger King, and having placed my order for a chicken sandwich and fries I was carrying two cups of ketchup to my table when my cell phone rang. I almost dropped my ketchup getting the phone off my belt. When I learned what the call was about, I almost dropped my teeth too (no, they're not removable). It was James Currie from the Pensacola Sports Association, the organization that in 2010 had honored five of us from the Florida Emerald Coast area, as related in chapter 15.

Mr. Currie informed me that the Association (PSA) had nominated me for Amateur Athlete of the Year for 2013, and he was hoping I would be able to attend the annual awards dinner on April 10th. I assured him I would be there (another of those automatic decisions), and said goodbye, still wondering how many categories they had, such as sport, age, gender, amateur vs. professional, etc. Our local newspaper, *The Daily News*, has an athlete of the week and year for football, baseball, basketball, track and field, wrestling, volleyball, soccer, golf and several other sports I don't recall. In all of these they have large schools, small schools, males, females, etc. I'm not aware of a geezer category in any of these sports. So with the only category restrictions the PSA had being amateur or professional, you can imagine how and why I felt so highly complimented, and more than mildly excited, about even being nominated and invited to the event.

The banquet was 49 days away, so I had plenty of time to hope and wonder. But exactly nine days later I received a letter telling me that I had been "Selected as Amateur Athlete of the Year." I kept looking for the word "nominated" but did not find it. We were enjoying a visit from the retired vice president of the college I had retired from, Dr. Jim Willis and his wife Sylvia. I had them read the brief letter, then Sandy read it, then I read it and re-read it. None of us found the word "nominated." It said "selected." Wow!!

Well, finally April 10, 2014 rolled around, and what a gala event the awards banquet was, at least for me and my family and friends. My brother, Walker, drove down from Memphis with our remaining sister, Jo. We had lost our eldest sister, Bobbie, in 1998, and Billie in 2013, 42 days after my Hall of

Fame party at Walker's house. Norman and Violet Meeker were there, and our close friend, Iris Lawrence, as were Dr. Jim and Sylvia Willis. Kelly Berry, Sandy's boss, was there with her husband, Jeff, and Ruth McKinon, my boss at Pensacola State College. Dr. Bill Spain, my dear friend and Doctor of Chiropractic, without whose help this might never have happened, had bought a ticket, but had quintuple (that's five) bypass surgery a few days before. So what did he do? He asked a good friend, Theo Baars, to come in his place. Mr. Baars fit right in with the group, and he didn't know any of us. That is a good friend.

There was another couple who were not there, yet they were there. Sound like double talk? I had met a young lad of age 11 or so at the track where I trained a few years back, who has all the skills and attitude of a future champion sprinter. He also later played on the high school football team, and just recently received a trophy from Pensacola State College where he is a freshman (and where I teach as adjunct) naming him the fastest student in the school. His name is Rickey Maltbia Jr., and he has a younger sister who is into the sport now, and she also is scoring wins. Their parents are usually at the track with them, and I just kinda developed a respect, admiration and fondness for the entire family. One day not long ago the father and I were having a conversation, and I posed the question "You're a man of the cloth, aren't you?" With such manners from the children and the family values they all share, that one was pretty easy. And I was right.

Anyway, the Maltbias were not going to be able to attend the ceremony, but shortly before we sat down for the meal, Pastor and Mrs. Maltbia sneaked into the room just long enough to bring me a card and a gift and congratulate me. Well, guess what! We had two tickets from someone who had to cancel, and Sandy and I began the arm twisting. Mrs. Maltbia was dressed well but Pastor Maltbia felt that he was not "dressed for such an occasion." Sandy and I won, and they stayed and enjoyed the meal and festivities.

There were about two dozen awards given out for special achievements – a few to teams, but the majority of them went to individuals. When they finally got around to the Athlete of the Year award, they projected a collage of pictures of me on the big screen, while the emcee read from my "brag sheet" that I had provided for them. As he announced my name and my age, before I could get completely out of my chair, about 450 people rose, cheering and clapping. Talk about a feeling of exhilaration, I was about to get misty-eyed. No ... I really did get misty-eyed.

One of the two men who presented me with the award, a beautifully carved wooden plaque, was Coach Pete Shinnick. Coach Shinnick is the man the University of West Florida has hired to put together a football program for their entry into the world of college football in 2016. Well, the coach turned out to be the keynote speaker for the evening. As he was introduced a little later, he walked up on the podium to the microphone, turned toward our tables, pointed at me, and said "Before I start, John Hurd, I just want to say that you are my kind of hero." Have you any idea the kind of chill a person gets when something like that happens?!? Then for the next 16 minutes he had that audience in the palm of his hand. If he can inspire a bunch of college football players like he inspired us that night, UWF should have one heck of a team.

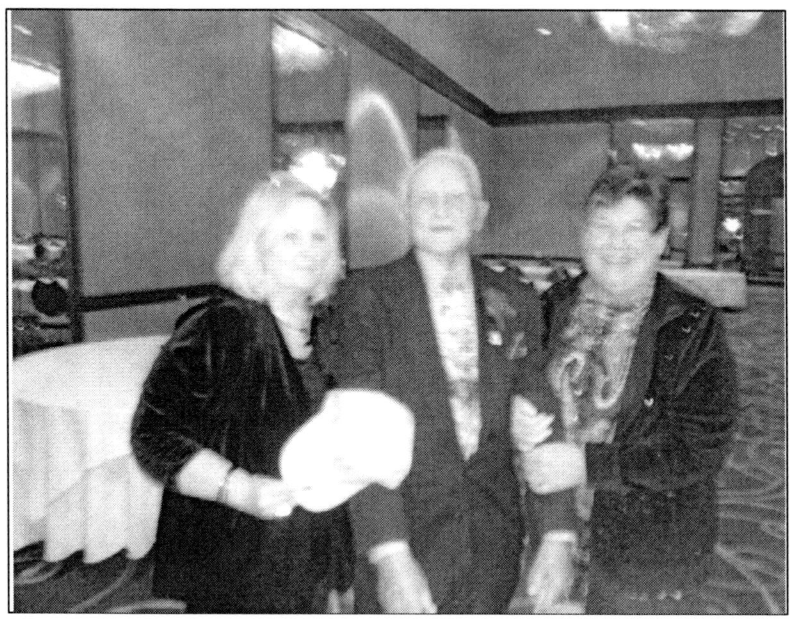

L to R: Jean and Edgar Buffaloe, and my bride Sandy Hurd at the induction of Edgar into The Memphis Amateur Sports Hall of Fame, boxing category, on December 2, 2013.

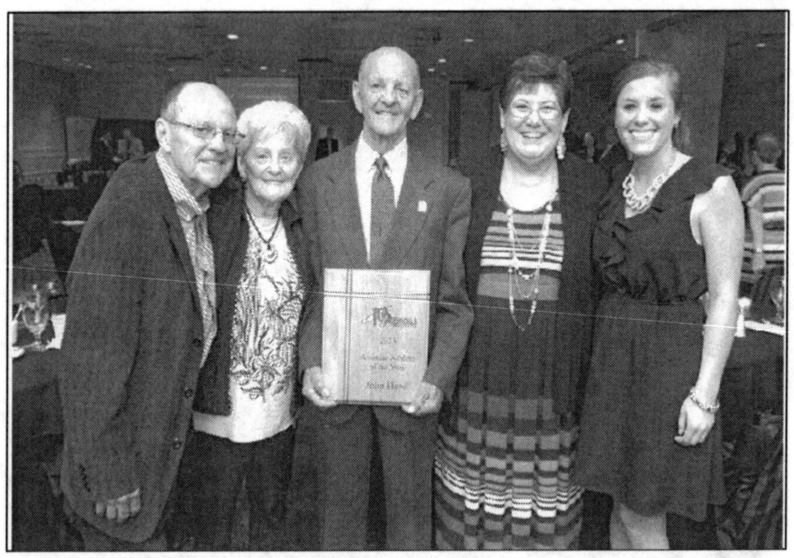

L to R: Walker Hurd, brother, Jo Lowery, sister, John Hurd, Sandy Hurd, wife, and Grier Halstead, PSA event coordinator, at the annual Pensacola Sports Association's award ceremony. John holds the plaque naming him Amateur Athlete of the Year 2013.

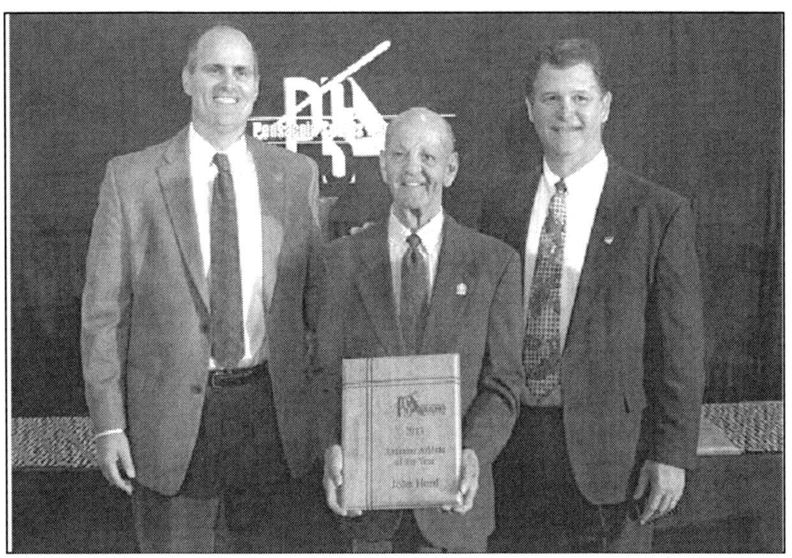

L to R: University of West Florida football coach Pete Shinnick, John Hurd, and Pensacola State College Athletic Director Bill Hamilton, at the annual Pensacola Sports Association's award ceremony.

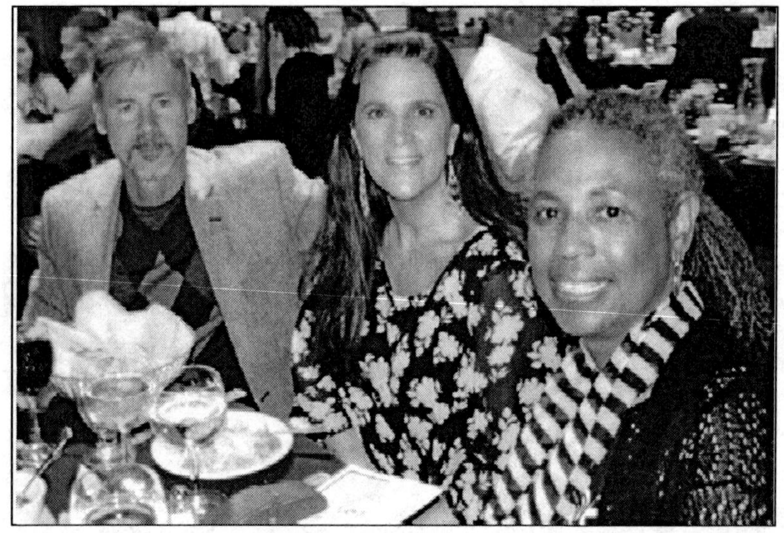

Jeff and Kelly Berry, Sandy's boss at Fisher Brown Bottrell Insurance, with Ruth McKinon, my boss at Pensacola State College (adjunct) at the PSA award ceremony.

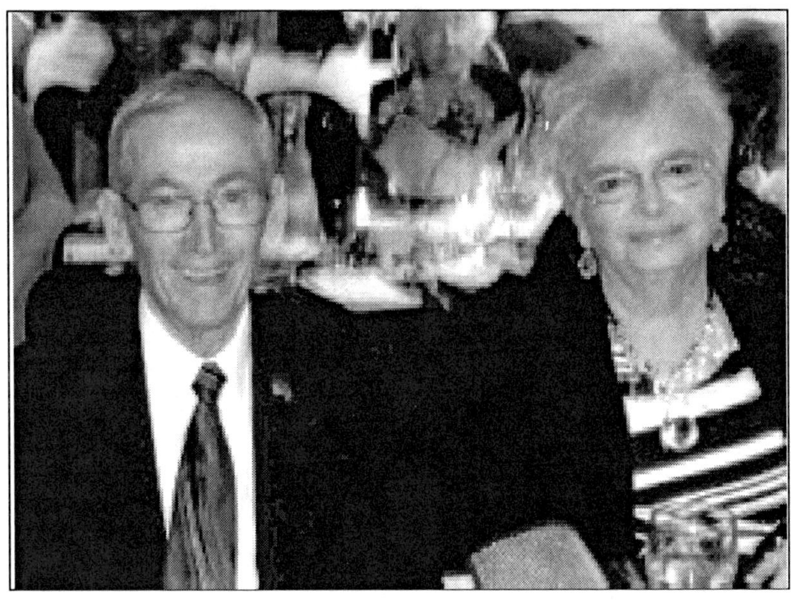

Sylvia and Jim Willis PhD, retired vice president of the college I retired from in Memphis as Associate Professor Emeritus, thanks to Jim, at the PSA award banquet in Pensacola, April 10, 2015.

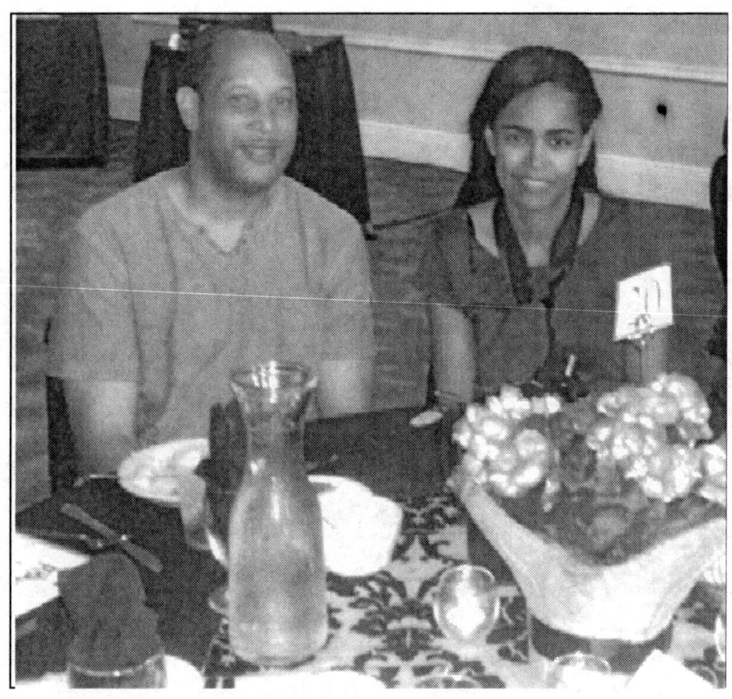

Pastor and Mrs. Rick Maltbia at the annual Pensacola Sports Association's award ceremony.

2014 FASTEST STUDENT ON CAMPUS

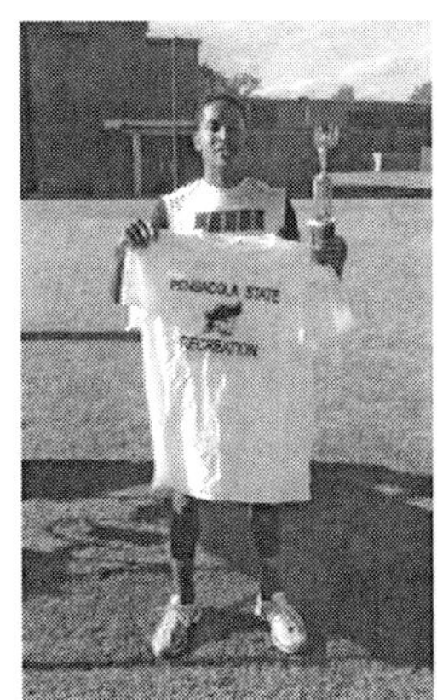

1st place winner

Rickey Maltbia

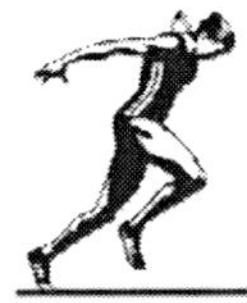

** Follow us on Facebook. Pensacola State Intramurals**

Rickey Maltbia, son of Pastor and Mrs. Maltbia, surely a future sprint champion, and all round young gentleman.

22
Has It Been Worth It?

In a word – ABSOLUTELY.

When I took up this sport just over 21 years ago at the age of 61, my hopes were to (A) improve my overall health, (B) get into better physical shape, (C) have some fun, (D) meet some new friends, and (E) maybe someday win a state gold medal.

(A) I've been fortunate enough to enjoy good health most of my life anyway. But I still feel that I'm as healthy as I was before I took up sprinting. And from age 61 to 83, most people would probably consider that in itself as an improvement, especially compared to the normal change most people experience at that stage of their lives.

Have I had injuries along the way? Sure. I've had both ankles sprained, an inflamed metatarsal, pulled a calf muscle, a hamstring muscle, and two groin muscles, and bruised or fractured a rib or two (the doctors were not sure). I have two heart conditions: mitral valve prolapse and left bundle branch block. But I had both of them before I began running, and the latter condition is believed to have been caused by a pharmacist's mixing up the labels on two prescription bottles in 1987.

Yes, I had some challenges with the dizzy spells, before learning what caused them. But, you know what? I probably had that out-of-alignment vertebra since birth. And I'm pretty sure that it was the major cause of the anxiety/panic attacks (agoraphobia) I endured for so many years. I can't prove it, of course, because I have no medical training. But I never met a doctor who had a clue what I was going through with the attacks, so I guess that makes us even. They want to attribute all of it to a state of mind, and of course much of it is related to that. But I contend that some physical change initially brought on that state of mind.

I cite two incidents to support that theory:

(1) One night, years ago, I was having a particularly tough time powering down to get to sleep. I was on my left side, and when I rolled over onto my right side, "it" instantly changed, totally, and I was perfectly relaxed. It was as if I had flipped the "off" switch when I rolled over.

(2) When I was about 55, I went through a series of ten sessions with a Rolfer. Rolfing has to do with breaking up the fascia that retains tension in your muscles and joints. When he reached deep into a certain point around mid-torso, I went into an instant state of high anxiety. He recognized it immediately for what it was, and eased off. In neither of these incidents did my mindset turn off or on by itself.

I do concede that after experiencing a few real panic attacks, they can be brought on by your thoughts. You begin to avoid places that will be confining. You will find yourself not going to a movie or even to church, or at least arrive early and get an aisle seat, and even refuse to move down for late comers when the usher asks you to make room for them. You might avoid the freeways, where exits may be far apart, or get on and stay in the right lane for a quick exit. In other words, you will do anything to avoid another episode. I believe it's not fear of the marketplace, as the name agoraphobia technically means; it's a fear of fear.

I endured them from 1948 till the mid-1960s. They returned in 1987, and I again went for professional help. During all that time, the terms anxiety or panic attack or hyperventilation were never used.

Have I been sick during those 21 plus years? I've had maybe two or three colds or sore throats, but nothing to visit a doctor for, or buy over the counter medicines. I recently had a test for free radicals, the things you might take antioxidants for. As it was explained to me, if your count is lower than 500 (whatever that means) it is good, from 500 to 750 is middle ground, and over 750 means you have issues. My count was 66, the lowest the testing doctor had ever seen. And, as I mentioned earlier, my average blood pressure reading over the last several years is 121/65.

(B) As for getting into shape: Having been issued at birth fast twitch (white, limited oxygen) muscles, I am anaerobic and still would have a tough time running a mile. But I recover quickly from my sprints, and that is what is required in my game. And my kind of training, high-intensity short bursts of power, is what increases the human growth hormone, as I learned from Phil

Campbell's book. Some people buy human growth hormone (HGH) at the drugstore.

(C) About having fun. I have a rule that I live by: If it isn't fun, I'll find something else to do. I've been sprinting for just over 21 years, and I'm having a ball. (Except for Sandy, I've never stayed with anything that long, even a job or a house to live in.)

(D) And I've made good friends everywhere I've been, at the practice track and at the games. Some of my best friends are the guys I compete with.

(E) Now, about someday maybe winning a gold medal for a state championship. So far I've accumulated 60 of them, and at the national level I have 6 golds, 2 silvers, and 9 ribbons (5th-8th).

I'm looking forward to seeing what it's going to be like, competing on the other side of age 100.

Highlights and Awards 1993-2014

Did not participate in track in school. Way too small.

In 1993 began competitive sprinting at age 61.

Have won state championships in Tennessee, Florida, Arkansas, Mississippi, Alabama, and Louisiana.

Participated in 67 individual events in and for Pensacola area and State of Florida. Won 66 gold medals and one silver medal.

Won State of Florida championships in both the 100 meter and 200 meter dashes for 10 consecutive years – 2003-2012. Both of those are unofficial state records. The next closest was one man who won one event for four consecutive years. Missed the state games in 2013 because of wife's illness. Won them again in 2014, along with the new 50 meter dash.

In 2007 National Senior Games won my first national medal, a gold one in the 4x100 meter relay.

In 2011 National Senior Games won silver in the 100 meter dash, silver in the 200 meter dash, and gold in the 4x100 meter relay.

In 2013 National Senior Games won gold in the 100 meter dash, gold in the 200 meter dash, gold in the 50 meter dash, and gold in the 4x100 meter relay. The latter two are American records.

In 2010 received a Pensacola Sports Association Special Achievement Award. Had won the Florida state gold medals for the 100 meter and 200 meter dashes for the seventh consecutive year, 2003-2009.

In 2012 inducted into the Memphis Amateur Sports Hall of Fame, track and field category.

In 2014 received the Pensacola Sports Association award for "Amateur Athlete of the Year for 2013." They have two categories for this award: amateur and professional. It covers all sports, genders and ages. Was 82 years old.

Earned All American recognition in 17 out of the last 18 years, 1997-2014. Missed in 2005 by 1/100th of a second.

Records held:	Florida – 200 meter dash for 75-79 age bracket - 32.66 seconds, December 2006
	Florida – 50 meter dash for 80-84 age bracket – 8.90 seconds, December 2012
	National – 50 meter dash for 80-84 age bracket 8.72 seconds, July 2013
	National – 4x100 meter relay for 80-84 age bracket. 75.99 seconds, July 2013
Medals Count:	Gold 112 Silver 41 Bronze 8

'IA information can be obtained
vw.ICGtesting.com
'd in the USA
'02n0918071216
'S